The Instant Pot
Whole30 Cookbook

The Ultimate Instant Pot Cookbook With 107 Quick, Easy and

Healthy Recipes for Your Instant Pot Pressure Cooker

Esther Rollins

CONTENTS

Introduction

There are so many reasons why you need to consider using the Instant pot whole30. These include the following;

#1: Instant pot saves time and energy

With instant pot, foods are cooked speedily, with the use of pressure-cooking methods. The instant cooker can reduce cooking time by as much as 70% when compared to other methods. Less water is used in this 100% insulated external water pot, and instant pot remain the best energy saving cooking appliance in the world today.

#2: Preserves nutrients and produce better tasting foods

Heat is distributed more evenly with instant pot cooking, hence the use of an instant pressure cooker in preparing the whole 30 recipes will ensure that nutrients are quickly and deeply distributed.
With instant pot, you don't have to immerse the food in water, the steam available is enough to distribute heat evenly and quickly and for these reason essential and vital nutrients such as minerals and vitamins are not leached into water.

Since the food are surrounded by steam from the instant pot, there will be no oxidation, hence the food can keep its original flavor. Electric pressure cooker makes use of a fully sealed cooking techniques, hence your delicate veggies such as broccoli, and asparagus, will retain their bright colours.

#3: Instant pot destroys harmful micro-organisms in food

With the aid of the instant pot pressure cooker, food is prepared at a temperature higher than the boiling point of water, and for this reason, all harmful micro-organisms are destroyed within the shortest period of time, and these include the pathogenic bacteria and parasites.

Instant pot pressure cookers have been used for decades as sterilizers, especially for jam pots as well as glass baby bottles. Instant pot Pressure cookers are also used in treating water.

Some food items can carry huge loads of aflatoxins, which are naturally occurring mycotoxins produced by numerous species of the fungi – Aspergillus. Many foods can develop mycotoxins due to improper storage conditions such as temperatures and humidity. Aflatoxins in food can trigger a number of diseases and infections, including liver cancer, especially when the food is not prepared very well. Aside from liver cancer, aflatoxins can trigger other problems such as diarrhea, constipation and general and slow functioning of the vital organs.

Heating foods to the boiling point will not destroy all aflatoxins because many of them possess strong resistance to heat. Researches conducted by some Korean researches have confirmed that the use of instant pot in heating food can reduce the concentration of aflatoxins to the safest levels.

When cooking the Mexican chili for instance, the kidney beans used in this recipe contains a huge concentration of aflatoxin, however, boiling these kidney beans at high temperatures in instant pot for about 10 minutes can actually cause the destruction of the aflatoxins.

Instant pot Whole 30 Breakfast Recipes

Recipe #1: Fried Venison back-strap

(Total time: 45 minutes, servings: 8)

Ingredients:

- 1 (lbs.) venison blackstrap, cut into ¼ inch thick slices,
- 2 cups of milk,
- 2 tablespoons of hot pepper sauce,
- 2 large eggs,
- ½ a cup of milk,
- 3 cup of all-purpose flour,
- 2 tablespoons of salt,
- 1 tablespoon of black pepper (ground),
- 3 cups of vegetable oil.

Directions

1. Get a shallow bowl and inside place the venison back-strap, then pour in the hot sauce and milk, stir for the venison to coat, and marinate for about an hour. Get a shallow bowl and inside whisk the eggs and milk. Get a separate bowl and inside stir together the flour, pepper and salt.
2. Mix everything together and add into the sauce pan, then secure the lid and valve before choosing the "Sauté" option and choose 25 minutes cooking time.
3. Once the cooking is completed, let the instant pot pressure releases itself automatically. Cool for few minutes before serving.

Calories: 115; Total fat: 17.9g, Carbs: 10.22g, Dietary fiber; 1.77g, Sugars 1.05g ; proteins 20.67g; Cholesterol 185mg; Sodium :266mg

Recipe #2: Goat Curry in a hurry

(Total time: 25 minutes, servings: 2)

Ingredients:

- 2 tablespoons of oil (avocado oil preferred),
- 2 lbs. of goat or lamb (bone-in-goat preferred),
- 2 diced onions,
- 1 ½ inch knob of minced fresh ginger, and
- 3 cloves of minced garlic, and
- 4 whole cloves or, a teaspoon of any spice of your choice

Directions

1. Press on the "sauté" button in the instant pot, then add the oil alongside the goat meat unto the pot. Add the onion, ginger, garlic and the spice once the meat begins to brown.
2. Pour in the remaining spice (if there is any left), then secure the lid and close the pressure valve. Cook for about 15 minutes.
3. Let the pressure releases itself naturally after cooking, and serve immediately.

Calories: 142; Total fat: 17.2g, Carbs: 7.9g, Dietary fiber; 1.8g, Sugars 1.1g ; proteins 16.35g; Cholesterol 190mg; Sodium :328mg

Recipe #3: The Chinese Broccoli recipe

(Total time: 25 minutes, servings: 4)

Ingredients:

- 1 lbs. of Broccoli,
- ¼ of a cup of butter or margarine,
- ¼ cup of water,
- 1 tablespoon of soy sauce,
- 1 tablespoon of soy sauce,
- 1 cup of celery (thinly sliced),
- 1 can of 5 ounce water chestnuts(sliced and drained),
- 1 ½ tablespoons of sesame seeds.

Directions

1. Trim out the outer leaves and ends of the broccoli, then cut the stalks and florets into 2-inch lengths before slicing lengthwise into halves.
2. Add the trimmed broccoli alongside other ingredients to the pan of the instant pot and close the lid before setting the high pressure and cooking time at 20 minutes. Make sure you choose "sauté" option on the instant pot.
3. Once the cooking time is completed, allow the pressure cooker to release itself (it should take about 10 minutes). Pour the broccoli recipe in a serving bowl.

Calories: 114; Total fat: 8.8g, Carbs: 5.45g, Dietary fiber; 4.7g, Sugars 1.01g ; proteins 16.3g; Cholesterol 174mg; Sodium :329mg.

Recipe #4: Knoephla soup

(Total time: 30 minutes, servings: 4)

Ingredients:

- 1 diced potato (large),
- 1 cup of celery (diced),
- 1 ½ cups of carrots (diced),
- ½ a bag of spätzle dumping,
- 2 cans of chicken soup ,
- 2 cups of chicken broth,
- ½ tablespoons each of pepper and salt.

Directions

1. Add all your ingredients except chicken soup into the instant pot, and cover with the lid before you close the pressure valve. Then set the time at 15 minutes at high pressure to cook the soup.
2. Slowly release the valves before you open the instant pot lid.
3. Serve immediately.

Calories: 151g; Total fat: 11.78g, Carbs: 12.9g, Dietary fiber; 6.7g, Sugars 5.4g ; proteins 9.68g; Cholesterol 118mg; Sodium :518 mg

Recipe #5: Instant pot deep-fry Pretzel coated fried fish

(Total time: 30 minutes, serving: 4)

Ingredients:

- 1 quart of oil,
- ¾ of a cup of all-purpose flour,
- 1 teaspoon of salt,
- ½ a teaspoon of ground black pepper,
- ¾ of a cup of crushed pretzels,
- 2 large eggs,
- 1 lb. of frozen cod fillets (thawed).

Directions

1. Spread the fish on a plate and then rob the flour on them.
2. Press the "Sauté" button on the instant pot and then add all ingredients along with the fish. Sauté for about 25 minutes under high pressure, and while the valve is tightly closed.
3. Release the valve and cool the deep-fried fish for about 2 minute before serving.

Calories: 89; Total fat: 8.79g, Carbs: 2.5g, Dietary fiber; 0.65g, Sugars 0.77g ; proteins 22.1g; Cholesterol 186mg; Sodium :442mg.

Recipe #6: The Instant pot sweet potato

(Total time: 25 minutes, servings: 4)

Ingredients:

- 1 cup of water,
- 4 medium to large sweet potatoes,

Directions

1. Place your steamer basket inside the instant pot and add the water. Scrub your sweet potatoes and make sure the skin are clean and then place the potatoes on the top of the steamer basket.
2. Cover the mix and place the vent on the instant pot lid to seal.
3. Set the instant pot at "steam" and set cooking time at 10 minutes.
4. Once the cooking is completed, do not be in a hurry to open lid, let the pressure reduce naturally (about 20 minutes).
5. Lift the lid and serve immediately

Calories: 192g; Total fat: 9.9g, Carbs: 12.6g, Dietary fiber; 4.5g, Sugars 8.34g ; proteins 7.8g; Cholesterol 114mg; Sodium :86mg

Recipe #7: Instant pot taco meat

(Total time: 25 minutes, servings: 2)

Ingredients:

- 2lbs. of ground beef,
- 4 tablespoons of olive oil,
- 2 red diced onions,
- 3 green diced bell peppers,
- 5 minced garlic cloves,
- 2 teaspoons of chili powder,
- 2 teaspoons of oregano,
- 1 teaspoon of salt,
- 1 teaspoon of basil (dried),
- ½ a teaspoon of turmeric,
- ½ a teaspoon of black pepper,
- 1 teaspoon of paprika,
- 1 teaspoon of cumin,
- ½ a teaspoon of cayenne,
- ½ a teaspoon of chipotle powder,
- Cilantro (for garnishing).

Directions

1. Add all ingredients (except the ground beef), into the instant pot, then press the "sauté" button and stir-fry for about 6 minutes.
2. Add the brown beef unto the pot and cook further for 2 minutes until it turns brown.
3. Secure the lid and then close the pressure valve and cook further for 10 minutes at high pressure.
4. Let the pressure release from the instant pot naturally, once the met is done cooking or simply perform the quick release option.
5. Open the lid and garnish with the cilantro when serving.

Calories: 146; Total fat: 21.2g, Carbs: 10.07g, Dietary fiber; 1.93g, Sugars 0.87g ; proteins 23.4g; Cholesterol 168mg; Sodium :331mg

Recipe #8: The delicious fried fish Tacos

(Total time: 45 minutes, servings: 10)

Ingredients:

- 1 cup of all-purpose flour,
- ½ a teaspoon of salt,
- 1 ½ lbs. of cubed cod fillets,
- 1 quart of vegetable oil,
- 20 corn tortillas (6 inch),
- 5 cups of shredded cabbage,
- 1 cup of mayonnaise,
- ¼ of a cup of salsa,
- 1 lime (cut into wedges).

Directions

1. Get a shallow bowl, and inside, whisk together the flour, and salt. Rinse the fish and pat it dry, then cut them into 10 equal pieces.
2. Add the mix into the instant pot pressure cooker alongside other ingredients. Close the lid, and set at sauté option before setting the cooking temperature at 25 minutes.
3. Once the cooking is done, simply allow the pressure to release naturally – this will take some 10 to 15 minutes, then gently un-lid the pot and pour the recipe into a serving bowl.

Calories: 108; Total fat: 15.87g, Carbs: 6.1g, Dietary fiber; 0.99g, Sugars 1.2g ; proteins 16.58g; Cholesterol 183mg; Sodium :284mg

Recipe #9: Deep-fried Butterfield Shrimp

(Total time: 35 minutes, servings: 4)

Ingredients:

- 1 lb. of large shrimp (peeled, deveined and butter-flied),
- 2 large eggs,
- 5 cup of oil (for deep frying),
- 2 cup of bread crumbs(fresh),
- 1 quart of water, and
- 1 ½ cup of corn starch.

Directions

1. Press the "sauté" button on the instant pot before adding the ingredients (except bread crumbs). Sauté for 10 minutes then press the "cancel" button
2. Add the bread crumbs before pressing the "deep fry" option on the instant pot and fry for about 15 minutes.
3. Serve immediately.

Calories: 175; Total fat: 16.9g, Carbs: 12.56g, Dietary fiber; 2.02g, Sugars 3.99g ; proteins 22.1g; Cholesterol 265mg; Sodium :417mg

Recipe #10: The Instant Pot Pineapple-Coconut-Lime Rice

(Total time: 33 minutes, serving: 4)

Ingredients:

- 1 ½ cups of uncooked long-grain white rice,
- 1 cup of water,
- 1 (8 ounce) of undrained crushed pineapple,
- ¾ of a cup of coconut milk,
- ¼ of a teaspoon of red pepper flakes,
- 1 lime (juiced and zested).

Directions

1. Rinse the water clearly and place the drained rice into the instant pot. Add the water and pineapple chunks alongside the juice, coconut milk, and red pepper flakes. Place the pot lid and lock it in place.
2. Turn on the instant pot and choose the manual setting and high pressure. Set the timer at 3 minutes and after cooking time, simply let the pressure release itself naturally (this will take about 20 minutes).
3. Stir in the lime zest and juice and serve.

Calories: 119; Total fat: 9.66g, Carbs: 14.06g, Dietary fiber; 2.45g, Sugars 7.4g ; proteins 13.38g; Cholesterol 92mg; Sodium :115mg.

Recipe #11: Gambas Pil-Pil (The Chilean Prawns)

(Total time: 32 minutes, servings: 6)

Ingredients:

- 10 cloves of garlic (slightly crushed and peeled),
- 3 tablespoons of brandy or pisco,
- ½ a teaspoon of salt,
- ½ a cup of grapeseed oil or olive oil,
- 1 ½ lbs. of large shrimp (de-veined and peeled),
- ½ teaspoon of cayenne pepper
- 1 Cacho de Cabra pepper (or Anaheim pepper), it must be seeded and cut into ½ inch pieces, and
- 1 lime (cut into wedges)

Directions

1. Get a bowl, and inside, place the garlic cloves and the grapeseed oil, and pour into the instant pot. Set the cooking time at 5 minutes at high pressure after covering the pot with lid and securing the valve. Cook until the garlic cloves turn golden brown, and the oil has become hot.
2. Add the remaining ingredients and set at "sauté" option and set cooking temperature at 15 minutes.
3. Make use of the quick release option after the cooking and pour into a serving bowl.

Calories: 79; Total fat: 1.9g, Carbs: 3.4g, Dietary fiber; 0.77g, Sugars 0.42g ; proteins 20g; Cholesterol 68mg; Sodium :433mg.

Recipe #12: The Low carb, Instant Pot Jamaican Jerk Pork Roast

(Total time: 50 minutes, servings: 12)

Ingredients:

- 4 lbs., of pork shoulder,
- ¼ of a cup of jerk spice blend (no sugar),
- 1 tablespoon of olive oil, and
- ½ a cup of beef stock or broth.

Directions

1. Rub the pork with olive oil before coating with the spice blend.
2. Set the instant pot to the "sauté" option, and brown the meet in all sides.
3. Add the broth, then seal the top of the Instant pot and cook at high pressure for 35 minutes.
4. Release the pressure of the instant pot after cooking, then shred and serve immediately.

Calories: 115; Total fat: 12.3g, Carbs: 3.9g, Dietary fiber; 0.96g, Sugars 0.45g ; proteins 23.4g; Cholesterol 106mg; Sodium :274mg

Recipe #13: The Instant pot double bean and Ham soup

(Total time: 1 hour 10 minutes, servings: 6)

Ingredients:

- 2 cups of navy beans (dry),
- 1 large onion (chopped)
- 2 cups of chicken broth,
- 2 stalks celery (chopped)
- 2 cups of water,
- 1 can (16 ounce) of pork and beans (undrained),
- 1 cup of chopped ham,
- 1 can (14.5 ounce), of undrained diced tomatoes,
- 2 large carrots(chopped), and
- ½ teaspoon each of salt and pepper

Directions

1. Add the navy beans alongside the chicken broth, carrots, onion, tomatoes, water and celery into the instant pot, then seal the pressure cooker and turn the knob to "sauté" and set the timer at 45 minutes.
2. Release the pressure manually when the timer is completed.
3. Remove the lid and stir the pork, beans and the ham, before you season with salt and pepper.

Calories: 152; Total fat: 19.8g, Carbs: 9.4g, Dietary fiber; 1.3g, Sugars 2g ; proteins 19.77g; Cholesterol 301mg; Sodium :341mg

Recipe #14: Ketogenic Instant pot Soup

(Total time: 58 minutes, serving: 6)

Ingredients:

- 1 tablespoon of olive oil,
- 1 yellow onion (diced),
- 2 cloves of minced garlic,
- 1 head of cauliflower (coarsely chopped),
- 1 green chopped bell pepper,
- 1 tablespoon of onion powder,
- ½ teaspoon each for salt and black pepper,
- 1 container (32 ounce) of chicken stock,
- 2 cups of shredded cheddar cheese,
- 1 cup of half-and –half,
- 1 tablespoon of Dijon Mustard,
- 4 dashes of hot pepper sauce.

Directions

1. Turn on the instant pot, and choose the "sauté" function. Add the olive oil and then the onion and garlic and sauté until brown- this should take about 3 minutes. Add the green bell pepper, alongside cauliflower onion powder, pepper and salt, then pour in the chicken stock and close the lid before selecting the "soup" function. Set the timer at 15 minutes.

2. Make use of the quick release option to release the pressure after cooking (this should take about 5 minutes). Unlock and take off the lid before adding the cheddar cheese, half-and-half, turkey bacon, hot sauce, and Dijon mustard. Select the "sauté" function again, and cook for about 5 minutes until it becomes bubbly.

Calories: 117; Total fat: 18.5g, Carbs: 9.4g, Dietary fiber; 2.62g, Sugars 1.34g ; proteins 21.7g; Cholesterol 285mg; Sodium :227mg

Recipe #15: The steamed artichoke

(Total time: 30 minutes, serving: 2)

Ingredients:

- 2 large , and whole artichokes,
- 1 garlic clove,
- 1 tablespoon of lemon juice, and
- 1 bay leaf

Directions

1. Cut and discard the stem of artichoke, and ensure the bottom of the artichokes are flat. Likewise, cut the top 1 inch of the artichokes and discard, and the thorny end of each artichoke leaves must be snipped with a scissors, and disposed.
2. Fill up the bottom of the instant pot with water, and add all the ingredients before adding the artichokes.
3. Place the artichoke inside the instant pot and choose "boil" option. Set the timer at 20 minutes at high pressure then place the lid and make sure the valves are seal. Let the instant pot release the pressure naturally once the cooking is done.

Calories: 87; Total fat: 3.6g, Carbs: 9.4g, Dietary fiber; 2.87g, Sugars 1.46g ; proteins 18.4g; Cholesterol 56mg; Sodium :117mg

(Total time: 35 minutes, serving: 2-4)

Ingredients:

- 2 lbs.
- 1 teaspoon of salt,
- ½ a teaspoon of black pepper,
- 4 cups of cauliflower,
- 1 medium onion (chopped),
- 4 cloves of garlic,
- 2 ribs of celery,
- 8 ounces of sliced Portabella mushrooms,
- 2 tablespoons of organic coconut oil and
- 2 cups of clean water.

Directions

1. Place the cauliflower alongside the onion, garlic, celery and water in the bottom of the instant pot. Top up with the pork and season with the salt and pepper.
2. Set the instant pot at boil option and cook at high pressure for 15 minutes after closing the pot and after sealing the valves.
3. Prepare the gravy while the pork is being prepared. Transfer the cooked veggies to the blender and blend smoothly.
4. Cook the mushroom along with the veggies in the instant cooker for 5 minutes (sauté option must be selected). Then serve the mushroom gravy on top of the Pork

Calories: 217; Total fat: 23.4g, Carbs: 11g, Dietary fiber; 3.8g, Sugars 4.2g ; proteins 26.2g; Cholesterol 305mg; Sodium :449mg

Recipe #17: The Sicilian stuffed artichoke

(Total time: 45 minutes, servings: 4)

Ingredients:

- 4 big artichokes,
- 4 garlic cloves,
- 2 tablespoons of olive oil,
- 1 fresh lemon (cut into wedges),
- 1 pinch of salt, and
- 8 ounces of thinly sliced Romano cheese.

Directions

1. Remove the stems and tops of the artichokes, then wiggle them back and forth with your thumbs in order to open the leaves. Gently snap off and remove the outer tougher leaves.
2. Place the lemon wedges inside a bowl of water to soak the artichokes (soak the artichokes for about 30 minutes).
3. Remove the artichokes from the water and shake off excess water from them. Insert the sliced Romano cheese in-between the artichoke leaves and then place a garlic clove in the center of each artichoke.
4. Place the artichoke inside the instant pot and choose "boil" option. Set the timer at 30 minutes at high pressure then place the lid and make sure the valves are seal. Let the instant pot release the pressure naturally once the cooking is done.

Calories: 102; Total fat: 5.8g, Carbs: 4.7g, Dietary fiber; 5.5g, Sugars 2.1g ; proteins 12.6g; Cholesterol 68mg; Sodium :285mg

Recipe #18: The Instant Pot Paleo Egg Roll Soup

(Total time: 40 minutes, serving: 4)

Ingredients:

- 1 teaspoon of olive , ghee or avocado oil,
- 1 lb. of ground organic pork,
- 1 diced large onion,
- 32 ounces (4 cups) of chicken or beef broth,
- ½ chopped head of cabbage,
- 2 cup of shredded carrots,
- 1 teaspoon of garlic powder,
- 1 teaspoon of onion powder,
- 1 teaspoon of sea salt,
- 1 teaspoon of ground ginger,
- 2/3 of a cup of coconut aminos, and
- 2 tablespoons of tapioca starch.

Directions

1. Brown the ground pork inside the instant pot with the oil, and onion. Cook until it is no longer pink (this should take 5 minutes).
2. Add the remaining ingredients and coo further for 20 minutes at high pressure, and once cooking is done, use the quick release option to release the pressure.
3. Remove the lid of the instant pot and serve immediately.

Calories: 120; Total fat: 17.49g, Carbs: 8.4, Dietary fiber;1.15g, Sugars 1.77g ; proteins 22.1g; Cholesterol 315mg; Sodium : 322mg.

Recipe #19: Instant Pot Mac and Cheese with Ham and Peas

(Total time: 44 minutes, serving: 6)

Ingredients:

- 4 cups of water,
- 1 pack (16 ounces) of elbow macaroni,
- 1 tablespoon of dry mustard powder,
- 1 teaspoon of salt,
- 1 tablespoon of hot sauce (optional),
- 1 can of evaporated milk (12 ounce),
- 1/3 of a cup of whole milk,
- 2 tablespoons of unsalted butter,
- 2 cups of shredded 2%milk cheddar cheese,
- 1 cup of shredded Monterrey Jack cheese,
- 1 cup of diced cooked ham,
- ½ cup of frozen peas (defrosted), and
- ½ a teaspoon each of salt and pepper (ground).

Directions

1. Add the water, with the macaroni, mustard powder, salt and hot sauce inside the instant pot. Close the pot and put the lid. Set the timer at 4 minutes, and set it at high pressure.

2. As the cooking is done, release the pressure slowly, with the aid of the quick release option. Unlock before removing the lid. Switch the function to low Sauté option by pressing the "sauté" once. Make sure you stir the macaroni to remove clumps.

3. Stir in the evaporated milk alongside the butter and milk into the pot. Add the cheddar and Monterrey cheese gradually and stir continuously until they become melted. Add the ham and peas before seasoning with salt and pepper.

Calories: 107; Total fat: 22.4g, Carbs: 12.14g, Dietary fiber; 2.02g, Sugars 7.4g ; proteins 20.1g; Cholesterol 228mg; Sodium :385mg.

Recipe #20: The Instant pot fall harvest pork soup (French onion soup)

(Total time: 1 hour 20 minutes, servings: 8)

Ingredients:

- 2 lbs. of boneless pork shoulder,
- 1 can of Campbell condensed French onion soup,
- ½ cup of apple cider,
- 3 large, cut Granny Smith apples,
- 3 cups of seeded, peeled and squash butternut,
- 2 medium peeled and cut parsnips,
- ½ teaspoon of dried and crushed thyme leaves.

Directions

1. Turn on the instant pot and set the timer at 35 minutes. Choose the "soup" option, and press high pressure.
2. Gently stir the pork, apples, cider, parsnips, soup, and thyme inside 5 quarts of water and add to the instant pot. Cover the mix and cook until the pork becomes tender. Press the release once the cooking is done and shred the pork before serving.

Calories: 89; Total fat: 22.13g, Carbs: 7.1g, Dietary fiber; 0.88g, Sugars 0.65g ; proteins 16.5g; Cholesterol 175mg; Sodium :287mg

Recipe #21: The Instant pot Thai Red Curry with Chicken

(Total time: 1 hour 12 minute, serving: 6)

Ingredients:

- 1 tablespoon of olive oil,
- ½ diced onion,
- 2 cloves of minced garlic,
- 1 stalk sliced celery,
- 6 large red potatoes (diced),
- ¾ cup of cherry tomatoes (diced),
- ½ a cup of chopped carrots,
- 2 boneless chicken breasts (sliced),
- 1 can (14 ounce) of coconut milk,
- 2 tablespoons of fish sauce,
- ½ a cup of water,
- ½ a cup of frozen peas,
- 3 tablespoons of red curry paste,
- 2 tablespoons of brown sugar,
- 3 chicken bouillon cubes (crushed).

Directions

1. Add the olive oil to the instant pot and put 'sauté' mode before heating the oil. Add the onion and garlic, then sauté further until they become soft (3 minutes). Add your celery and cook further until they turn bright green. Add the potatoes, along with the tomatoes and carrots and stir.
2. Place the chicken slices on top of the sautéed veggies, then pour the coconut milk on top of the chicken then add the fish sauce before you allow the liquid to boil (5 minutes). Mix in the water, peas, brown sugar, curry paste, and bouillon cubes.
3. Place the lid on the instant pot, and bring it to high pressure. Cook further for 12 minutes and release the pressure manually once the cooking time is reached.
4. Service immediately

Calories: 141; Total fat: 17.2g, Carbs: 11.38g, Dietary fiber; 3.04g, Sugars 4.23g ; proteins 24.01g; Cholesterol 271mg; Sodium : 388mg

Recipe #22: The Honey spiced Cajun Chicken

(Total time: 25 minutes, serving: 8)

Ingredients:

- 10 oz. of pounded chicken breast,
- Cooked linguini,
- 3 sliced large mushrooms,
- A diced large tomato,
- 2 tablespoons of mustard,
- 4 tablespoons of honey, and
- 3 .oz. of cream

Directions

1. Pat the chicken inside the seasonings.
2. Power on the instant pot and add the chicken, alongside all other ingredients into the pan. Close the lid and secure the valves and set the timer at 20 minutes. Make sure you select "sauté" option.
3. Once the time has lapsed, simply allow the instant pot to ease the pressure manually, and transfer the chicken into a serving bowl or plate.

Calories: 175; Total fat: 16.9g, Carbs: 12.56g, Dietary fiber; 2.02g, Sugars 3.99g ; proteins 22.1g; Cholesterol 265mg; Sodium :417mg

Recipe #23: The Instant pot mushroom Risotto

(Total time: 50 minutes, serving: 4)

Ingredients:

- ¼ of a cup of unsalted butter,
- ¼ of a cup of olive oil,
- 3 cup of diced mushrooms,
- 1 cup of chopped onion,
- 1 sprig of rosemary,
- 1 ½ cups of Arborio rice,
- 1 quart of a chicken stock,
- ½ of a cup of grated Parmesan cheese, and
- ½ teaspoon each of salt and pepper.

Directions

1. Press the "sauté" function on the instant pot, and then add the butter along with the olive oil. Stir for about 2 minutes until the butter melts, then add the mushroom and cook further while stirring occasionally (3 minutes). Stir in your onion and cook for extra 2 minutes, then add the rosemary sprig before cooking for 1 minute further.
2. Stir the rice into the pot and let them be coated with the butter and olive mix. Simmer for about 3 minutes before you pour the chicken stock, then stir to scrape the sides of the pot before you simmer again for 1 minute.
3. Close the lid and lock it, then turn on the venting knob at "sealed". Choose the manual function and set timer at 6 minutes. Choose high pressure.
4. Tap on the venting knob occasionally with a spatula or wooden spoon, then stand back and turn the knob to point at the vent. Remove the lid once the pressure has been released (5 minutes).
5. Stir the Risotto for about 1 minute, until it becomes creamy, then remove the rosemary sprig. Season with the salt and pepper before stirring in the parmesan cheese.

Calories: 156; Total fat: 12.6g, Carbs: 3.8g, Dietary fiber; 3.3g, Sugars 0.87g ; proteins 19.3g; Cholesterol 138mg; Sodium :175mg

Recipe #24: The Fish Batter with "Newcastle" Brown Ale

(Total time: 35 minutes, serving: 4)

Ingredients:

- ½ a teaspoon of garlic powder,
- ½ teaspoon of ground cinnamon,
- 1 qt. of vegetable oil for deep frying,
- ½ a cup of flour,
- ½ a cup of cornmeal,
- 1 teaspoon of garlic salt,
- 1 lb. of cod fillets (cut in pieces),
- 1 cup of brown ale (Newcastle brown ale).

Directions

1. Fry the vegetable oil inside the instant pot for 5 minutes, then whisk together the ingredients inside a large bowl and mix in your   until there are no lumps in the batter. Dip the fish cod inside the batter before you place them carefully in the instant pot.
2. Choose the "cook" option and high pressure. Set the timer at 25 minutes and wait until the cod become crispy and brown, especially at the sides.

Calories: 107; Total fat: 14.9g, Carbs: 7.5g, Dietary fiber; 1.7g, Sugars 0.9g ; proteins 19.4g; Cholesterol 174mg; Sodium :209mg

Recipe #25: The Bramboracky (Czech savory potato recipe)

(Total time: 60 minutes, serving: 3)

Ingredients:

- 4 medium to large potatoes,
- 2 large eggs,
- 3 cloves of crushed garlic,
- 1 tablespoon of milk,
- ½ teaspoon of salt ,
- ½ teaspoon of pepper,
- 3 tablespoons of all-purpose flour,
- 1 pinch of dried marjoram (optional),
- 2 teaspoons of olive oil , and
- 2 teaspoons of caraway seeds (optional)

Directions

1. Peel the potatoes and the grate them coarsely (make sure you squeeze out as much liquid as you can), put the shredded potato inside a bowl, and stir in your crushed garlic pepper, marjoram, salt, and caraway seeds. Get new bowl, and inside, beat the egg inside alongside the milk, then add the egg mix to the potatoes, before stirring well to combine. Mix in the flour gradually to form a thick but slurry batter.

2. Add the olive oil into the pan of the instant pot, and add the slurry batter. Set the option at "fry" and choose high pressure, then close the lid as well as the valve and press 25 minutes as the cooking time. Fry the pancake until they become golden brown in colour.

3. Once the frying time is completed, simply allow the instant pot to eject the pressure by itself (this may take up to 20 minutes). You can test the pancakes for doneness.

Calories: 78; Total fat: 11.4g, Carbs: 9.87g, Dietary fiber; 2.0g, Sugars 1.8g ; proteins 12.55g; Cholesterol 106mg; Sodium :325mg

Recipe #26: Savoy Cabbage with cream sauce

(Total time: 19 minutes, serving 4-6)

Ingredients:

- 1 cup of diced bacon or lardons,
- 1 large chopped onion,
- 2 cup of bone broth,
- 1 medium size head choy cabbage (finely chopped),
- ¼ of a teaspoon of mace (or nutmeg),
- ½ a can of coconut milk (200 mls),
- 1 bay leaf,
- ½ teaspoon of salt ,
- 2 tablespoons of parsley flakes.

Directions

1. Press the "sauté" option on the instant pot, and let the inner pot heat up. Add the bacon and onion, until they become crispy and lightly brown. Add the bone broth, then scrape the bottom of the pot to remove any stuck brown bits.
2. Stir in the cabbage and bay leaf, then cover with parchment round paper before you put the lid on top and then set the sealing valve to "sealing". Choose "manual" and then set cooking time at 4 minutes.
3. Once the cooking time has been reached, simply press the "keep warm/cancel", and then release the pressure before uncovering the pot and removing the parchment paper.
4. Press "sauté" again and add the nutmeg and coconut oil to boil. Simmer for 5 minutes before turning off the instant pot. Stir in the parsley flakes before serving.

Calories: 95; Total fat: 8.9g, Carbs: 7.4g, Dietary fiber; 4.2g, Sugars 1.04g ; proteins 13.7g; Cholesterol 137mg; Sodium :239mg

Recipe #27: Fried Teriyaki chicken wings

(Total time: 30 minutes, serving: 10-20)

Ingredients:

- 1/3 cup of lemon juice,
- ¼ cup of soy sauce,
- ¼ cup of vegetable oil,
- 3 tablespoons of chili sauce,
- A clove of finely chopped garlic,
- ¼ teaspoon of pepper,
- ¼ teaspoon of celery seed,
- A dash of mustard, and
- 3 pounds (15-20) chicken wings

Directions

1. Prepare the marinade by combining the lemon juice with soy sauce, chili sauce, oil, celery, garlic, pepper, and mustard. Stir very well and set aside.
2. Cut the chicken wings at the joint and remove the tips, then place the chickens in a dish.
3. Pour the marinade over chicken, and then refrigerate overnight, then drain before placing on broiler tray. Choose the "broil" option on the instant pot and set timer at 20 minutes. Once boiling is done, make sure you check the chicken for doneness before transferring them unto the plate.

Calories: 157; Total fat: 16.9g, Carbs: 8.33g, Dietary fiber; 1.3g, Sugars 2.1g ; proteins 21.9g; Cholesterol 196mg; Sodium :263mg

Instant pot Whole 30 Lunch Recipes

Recipe #28: The Instant pot baked beef soup

(Total time: 60 minutes, serving: 8)

Ingredients:

- 14 ounces of diced canned tomatoes (inside liquid),
- 1 cup of water,
- 3 tablespoons of tapioca,
- 2 tablespoons of sugar (preferably brown),
- ½ a teaspoon of pepper,
- 1 ½ teaspoons of salt,
- ½ a teaspoon of pepper,
- 2 lbs. of stew meat (cut into an inch cubes),
- 4 large carrots (diced into an inch chunks),
- 3 peeled and quartered potato,
- 2 celery ribs (cut into ¾ chunks),
- 1 large onion cut into smaller chunks, and
- A sliced bread.

Directions

1. Get a large bowl and combine the water with tomatoes, tapioca, salt, sugar and pepper. Add the remaining ingredients and mix properly.
2. Pour the mix into the instant pot and secure the lid and the valves before setting the cooking time at 30 minutes and choose "soup" option.
3. The vegetables should be tender and the soup becomes bubbly by the time the cooking has been completed. Let the pressure eases off naturally (this should take about 10 minutes).

Calories: 114; Total fat: 9.72g, Carbs: 4.8g, Dietary fiber; 0.79g, Sugars 0.45g ; proteins 9.5g; Cholesterol 168mg; Sodium :228mg

Recipe #29: Instant pot cooker Italian beef

(Total time: 2 hours 10 minutes, servings 2-4)

Ingredients:

- 3 lb. of organic chuck roast,
- 6 cloves of garlic,
- 2 teaspoons of garlic powder,
- 1 teaspoon of onion powder,
- ½ a teaspoon of ground ginger,
- 1 teaspoon of oregano,
- 1 teaspoon of basil,
- 1 teaspoon of marjoram,
- 1 teaspoon of sea salt ,
- 1 cup of beef broth, and
- ¼ of a cup of apple cider vinegar.

Directions

1. With the aid of a sharp knife simply cut some slits into the roast and then stuff them with garlic cloves.
2. Get a bowl and inside, simply whisk the organic powder with the onion, oregano, basil, ground ginger, marjoram, and salt and combine them well. Rub the seasoning blends on all sides of the roast, and place it inside the instant pot.
3. Pour the beef broth and apple cider vinegar into the pot before sealing the lid and ensure that the valve is closed.
4. Press the manual button and set cooking time at 90 minutes. Once the cooking is completed, simply allow the natural release to offload the pressure.
5. Remove the beef from the instant pot and shred with a fork.

Calories: 302; Total fat: 27.9g, Carbs: 13.9g, Dietary fiber; 4.18g, Sugars 2.9g ; proteins 28.6g; Cholesterol 325mg; Sodium :324mg

(Total time: 60 minutes, serving: 8)

Ingredients:

- 3 teaspoons of vegetable oil,
- 3 ½ cups of vegetable broth,
- 1 coarsely chopped onion,
- 4 cups of water,
- 2 thinly sliced shallots,
- 2 optional tablespoons of vegetarian fish sauce,
- 2 cloves chopped garlic,
- 2 tablespoons of red pepper flakes,
- 2-inch thinly sliced fresh ginger root,
- 1 bay leaf,
- 1 stalk of lemon grass (cut into 2-inch pieces),
- 2 kaffir lime leaves,
- 3 tablespoons of curry powder,
- 8 quartered small potatoes,
- 1 coarsely chopped green pepper,
- 1 can of coconut milk ,
- 2 peeled and sliced carrots,
- 2 cups of fresh bean sprouts(for garnishing),
- 8 sliced mushrooms,
- 8 sprigs of chopped cilantro(for garnishing),
- 1 lb. of pound tofu (cut into bit sizes).

Directions

1. Sauté the onion and shallots inside the sauce pan for 5 minutes until they become translucent and soft. Stir in your garlic, curry powder, lemon grass and ginger. Cook the mix for about 5 minutes, before stirring in the green pepper, mushrooms, carrots and tofu.

2. Pour the vegetable stock and water before seasoning with fish sauce and red pepper flakes. Bring the mix to boil before stirring in potatoes and coconut

milk.

3. Return the soup to boiling before reducing the heat to very low, to simmer- this should take about 20 minutes until the potatoes become tender. Garnish the bowl with cilantro and bean sprouts.

Calories: 210; Total fat: 17.1g, Carbs: 11.35g, Dietary fiber; 1.06g, Sugars 0.99g ; proteins 21.4g; Cholesterol 180mg; Sodium :218mg

Recipe #31: The family-friendly Amish chicken and corn soup

(Total time: 30 minutes, serving: 6)

Ingredients:

- 2 quarts of chicken stock or broth,
- ¼ cup of coarsely chopped onion
- ½ of stewing hen or fowl,
- ½ cup of coarsely chopped carrot,
- ½ cup of coarsely chopped celery,
- 1 teaspoon of saffron threads,
- ¾ of a cup of corn kernels,
- 1 teaspoon of chopped parsley (fresh),
- 1 cup of cooked egg noodles

Directions

1. Combine the stewing hen with the chicken stock, onion, carrot, celery, and saffron threads, and then bring to simmer inside the instant pot for 10 minutes at high pressure.
2. Remove the stewing hen mix and let it cool a bit, then separate the meat from the bone and cut into nice pieces. With the aid of a fine sieve, strain the saffron broth, and add the celery, corn, parsley and cooked noodles to your broth and return to instant pot and cover with the lid before you close the pressure valve. Then set the time at 10 minutes at high pressure again.
3. Serve immediately.

Calories: 169g; Total fat: 14.2g, Carbs: 13.1g, Dietary fiber; 6.9g, Sugars 3.67g ; proteins 13.88g; Cholesterol 279mg; Sodium :433mg

Recipe #32: The Japanese style deep-fried Shrimp

(Total time: 25 minutes, serving: 4)

Ingredients:

- 1 lb. of medium size shrimps (de-veined),
- ½ a teaspoon of salt,
- ½ a teaspoon of ground black pepper,
- ½ a teaspoon of garlic powder,
- 1 cup of all-purpose flour,
- 1 teaspoon of paprika,
- 2 large eggs (beaten),
- 1 cup of panko crumbs,
- 1 quart of olive oil.

Directions

1. Prepare the shrimp by removing unwanted items and then wash in water and leave for 3 minutes to dry.
2. Press the "sauté" button on the instant pot, and add the oil alongside other ingredients to the pot. Stir fry the mix for about 15 minutes and serve immediately.

Calories: 104; Total fat: 8.75g, Carbs: 5.4g, Dietary fiber; 1g, Sugars 0.79g ; proteins 12.6g; Cholesterol 89mg; Sodium :366mg

Recipe #33: The Ground beef chili

(Total time: 35 minutes, serving: 10)

Ingredients:

- 2lbs. ground beef,
- 2 tablespoons of olive oil,
- 2 diced red onions,
- 10 minced garlic cloves,
- 8 chopped carrots,
- 5 stalks of chopped celery,
- 2 chopped bell peppers,
- 1-2 minced jalapenos (remove the ribs and seeds),
- 4 cans of organic diced tomatoes,
- 2 teaspoons of chili powder,
- 1 tablespoon of cumin,
- 1 tablespoon of oregano,
- 2 tablespoon of salt,
- 1 teaspoon of black pepper, and
- ¼ of a teaspoon of cayenne.

Directions

1. Press the "sauté" button on the instant pot before adding the oil, garlic and onions. Sauté for a minute and add the ground beef and cook further until it becomes brown.
2. Add the other ingredients to the pot, and cover to lock the grid.
3. Simply press the "Keep warm/cancel" button, and then press the "bean/chili" button to tart the pressure cooking. This will be automatically set at 30 minutes (make sure you have closed the steam valve before cooking).
4. Once the chili has been prepared, the instant pot will switch automatically to the "Keep warm" mode. Do not use the quick release option, after cooking, simply allow the pressure to release itself naturally.
5. Garnish the meal with cilantro or sour cream.

Calories: 202; Total fat: 18.23g, Carbs: 9.15g, Dietary fiber; 4.3gg, Sugars 1.66g ; proteins 21.6g; Cholesterol 295mg; Sodium :379mg

Recipe #34: Scintillating Fried squid with Pineapple

(Total time: 25 minutes, serving: 4)

Ingredients:

- 4 stalks of celery (cut into 2 inch pieces),
- 2 tablespoons of vegetable oil,
- 3 cloves of minced garlic,
- 3 tablespoons of fish sauce,
- 1 large onion (cut into wedges),
- 1 teaspoon of brown sugar,
- 2 lbs. of squid (cleaned and sliced into ½ inch rings),
- 1/2 teaspoon of ground black pepper

Directions

1. Add the vegetable oil to the instant pot and press the "sauté" button, then sauté the garlic, until the garlic turns golden brown. Add the onion and stir-fry for about 60 seconds, then add the squid and cook further for 15 minutes until the squid turns white. Add the remaining ingredients and stir fry further for 2 minutes.

2. Once the cooking time is completed, simply allow the recipes to cool before serving.

Calories: 78; Total fat: 17.2g, Carbs: 10.6g, Dietary fiber; 1.19g, Sugars 0,66g ; proteins 18.71g; Cholesterol 118mg; Sodium :159mg

Recipe #35: Artichokes with sautéed navy beans

(Total time: 25 minutes, serving: 4)

Ingredients:

- 1 can of marinated artichoke hearts (quartered and drained),
- 6 tablespoons of olive oil,
- 2 minced garlic cloves,
- ½ teaspoon of freshly ground black pepper,
- ½ a teaspoon of salt , for added taste,
- ½ a teaspoon of ground red pepper,
- 1 can (15 ounces) of rinsed and drained navy beans,
- ¼ of a cup of grated Romano cheese

Directions

1. Heat olive oil inside the instant pot for about 5 minutes, and stir in the red pepper and garlic. Mix in the beans and continue cooking until it becomes crispy. Mix in your artichoke hearts and then cook further for about 2 minutes before seasoning with the black pepper.

2. Top up with Romano cheese before serving.

Calories: 92; Total fat: 16.9g, Carbs: 12.56g, Dietary fiber; 2.02g, Sugars 0.8g ; proteins 20.05g; Cholesterol 174mg; Sodium :266mg

Recipe #36: Instant pot stir fries with beef and green beans

(Total time: 30 minutes, serving: 4)

Ingredients:

- 1 clove minced garlic,
- 2 ½ tablespoons of vegetable oil,
- ¼ of a teaspoon of ground black pepper,
- ½ thinly sliced onion,
- 1 teaspoon of corn starch,
- 2 cups of fresh green beans (trimmed and washed),
- 1 teaspoon of vegetable oil,
- ¼ cup of chicken broth,
- 1 lb. of thinly sliced Sirloin tips, and
- 1 teaspoon of soy sauce.

Directions

1. Get a large mixing bowl and inside combine the black pepper with the garlic, cornstarch, and the vegetable oil. Add the beef and mix well. Then add the meat before cooking and stirring them for about 2 minutes inside the instant pot, until the beef has begun turning brown. Transfer the beef into a large bowl and then set it aside.
2. Add the onion and stir fry until it turns tender. Mix in the green beans and the broth, then cover and simmer for about 5 minutes until the beans have become crispy tender. Stir in your soy sauce plus the beef and cook while stirring continuously for about 2 minutes until the mix has been heated through.
3. Let the instant pot release the pressure once cooking is completed and serve immediately.

Calories: 101; Total fat: 15.2g, Carbs: 7.5g, Dietary fiber; 1.02g, Sugars 0.86g ; proteins 14.3g; Cholesterol 118; Sodium :186mg

Recipe #37: The chicken and veggie Miso soup

(Total time: 1 hour 7 minutes, servings: 7)

Ingredients:

- 1 -2 tablespoons of grapeseed oil,
- 5 carrots (chopped),
- 2 diced leeks,
- 5 ounces of shiitake mushrooms (sliced),
- 1 large onion (diced),
- 2 lbs. of skinless and boneless chicken thighs,
- ½ a teaspoon of salt and ground black pepper,
- 8 cups of chicken broth,
- ½ a cup of miso paste,
- 8 cloves of minced garlic,
- 1 tablespoon of soy sauce,
- 1 piece (2 inch) grated ginger root,
- 1 dash of sriracha. sauce
- ½ of a head of Napa cabbage (torn it to pieces),
- 1 head of a baby bok choy

Directions

1. Pour the grapeseed oil into the instant pot cooker, then add the carrots, leeks, shiitake mushrooms and onion. Select "sauté" setting and cook for 5 minutes.
2. Get a bowl and inside, season the chicken with salt and pepper, then add to the cooker and pour the chicken broth. Seal and cook after choosing the "soup" setting, and 7 minutes cooking time. Release the pressure manually after 10 minutes, then cover the vent with a dish towel before using the quick-release method.
3. Remove the chicken and shred with the aid of a fork, on a cutting board. Return the chicken to the cooker and add the miso paste, alongside the soy sauce, garlic, ginger and sriracha sauce. Cook further and stir while switching to "sauté" setting, until the miso paste ha dissolve completely (this should take some 5 minutes). Stir in your cabbage and the bok choy and cook further for 5 minutes until the whole recipe softens.

Calories: 156; Total fat: 17.38g, Carbs: 9.99g, Dietary fiber; 1.65g, Sugars 0.97g ; proteins 23.04g; Cholesterol 193mg; Sodium :428mg

Recipe #38: Instant pot shredded chicken

(Total time: 25 minutes, serving: 2-3)

Ingredients:

- 4 lbs. of chicken breast,
- ½ cup of water (or chicken broth),
- 1 teaspoon of salt, and
- ½ a teaspoon of black pepper.

Directions

1. Add all your ingredients into the instant pot, and cover with the lid before you close the pressure valve. Then set the time at 20 minutes at high pressure.
2. Once the cooking time has been completed, simply turn the instant pot's valve from sealing to venting for a quick release of pressure hence the steam will escape and you will be able to open the lid sooner.
3. Place the chicken on the cutting board and make use of forks to shred.
4. Store the chicken inside air-tight container alongside the cooking liquid to keep the meat moist.

Calories: 175; Total fat: 16.9g, Carbs: 12.56g, Dietary fiber; 2.02g, Sugars 3.99g ; proteins 22.1g; Cholesterol 265mg; Sodium :417mg

Recipe #39: The Instant pot Chickpea curry

(Total time: 35 minutes, serving: 8)

Ingredients:

- 2 tablespoons of vegetable oil,
- 2 minced average onions,
- 2 cloves of minced garlic,
- 2 tablespoons of fresh finely chopped fresh ginger root,
- 6 whole cloves,
- 2 sticks of crushed cinnamon ,
- 1 teaspoon of ground cumin,
- 1 teaspoon of ground coriander,
- ½ teaspoon of salt,
- ½ teaspoon of Cayenne pepper,
- 1 teaspoon of ground turmeric,
- 2 cans of garbanzo beans,
- 1 cup of fresh chopped cilantro

Directions

1. Open the instant pot and set it at "sauté". Heat the oil in the frying pan over and fry the onions until tender. Stir all other ingredients inside the oil and cook for about a minute while stirring constantly.
2. Mix the beans along with the liquid, and continue to cook the mix until all ingredients are blended (20 minutes).
3. Stir in the Cilantro once the cooking time is completed and you have released the valve.
4. Serve immediately.

Calories: 115; Total fat: 12.2g, Carbs: 9.6g, Dietary fiber; 2g, Sugars 1.5g ; proteins 19.7g; Cholesterol 144mg; Sodium :318mg

Recipe #40: The country chicken stew

(Total time: 40minutes, serving: 4)

Ingredients:

- 2 slices of diced bacon,
- 3 medium potatoes (cut into 1 inch pieces),
- A medium sliced onion,
- 2 medium sliced carrots,
- 1 condensed cream of chicken soup,
- 1 cup of frozen beans,
- 2 chunks of drained chicken breast in water,
- A can of soup water
- ½ teaspoon of crushed dried oregano leaves ,
- 2 tablespoons of fresh parsley (chopped).

Directions

1. Cook the bacon inside the instant pot with a little water, for 10 minutes at high pressure until it becomes crispy.
2. Remove the bacon and dry on paper towel. Add the onion inside the pot, and stir occasionally. Stir in the soup, oregano, carrots, and potatoes, then heat until the mix boils. Add the bacon into the pot again, cover to cook for about 15 minutes.
3. Stir in your beans, then cover and cook for about 10 minutes until the vegetable becomes tender. Stir in your parsley, bacon and chicken, then stir until the mixture becomes hot and bubbling.

Calories: 164; Total fat: 16.9g, Carbs: 12.56g, Dietary fiber; 1.7g, Sugars 2.3g ; proteins 22.6g; Cholesterol 215; Sodium :255mg

Recipe #41: Artichoke Salsa

(Total time: 15 minutes, serving: 5)

Ingredients:

- 1 jar (6.5 ounce) of drained and chopped , marinated artichoke hearts,
- 1 tablespoon of chopped garlic,
- 2 tablespoons of chopped fresh basil,
- ½ teaspoon each of salt and pepper (for added taste),
- 3 Roma Plum tomatoes (chopped),
- 2 tablespoons of chopped red onion, and
- ¼ of a cup of chopped black olives.

Directions

1. Get a medium size bowl and inside, mix all the ingredient and serve chilled under room temperature with Tortilla chip
2. To keep it warm, simply pour the recipe inside the instant pot and press "warm" and set the timer at 10 minutes and shut the valve after closing the lid.

Calories: 75; Total fat: 20.9g, Carbs: 14.36g, Dietary fiber; 3.7g, Sugars 6.04g ; proteins 19.5g; Cholesterol 175mg; Sodium :314mg

Recipe #42: The traditional instant pot Pho Ga Soup

(Total time: 30 minutes, serving: 5)

Ingredients:

- 1 tablespoon of vegetable oil,
- 2 shredded and cooked chicken breasts,
- 1 small chopped yellow onion,
- 4 green chopped onions,
- 1 pack baby bella mushroom (chopped),
- 1/3 of a cup of chopped fresh Cilantro,
- 4 minced garlic cloves,
- 2 cups of bean sprouts,
- 7 teaspoons of chicken bouillon
- 8 cups of water,
- 1 lime (sliced into wedges),
- 1 pack of rice stick noodles (about 7 ounces), and
- 1 dash of Sriracha hot sauce.

Directions

1. Sauté the onions, alongside the mushroom, and garlic and the veggies for about 10 minutes, until they become tender, inside the instant pot.
2. Add the water, alongside the rice noodles, as well as chicken bouillon, to the onion mix, and bring the mix to boil.
3. Mix the shredded chicken with the Cilantro, and green onions into the soup. Let the mix simmer for about 5 minutes, before transferring the soup inside the serving bowls. Top up with bean sprouts plus a squeeze of lemon juice as well as Sriracha sauce. And sauté for about 5 minutes, before the pressure cooker turns off.
4. Serve immediately.

Calories: 95; Total fat: 12.1g, Carbs: 6.77g, Dietary fiber; 4.1g, Sugars 1.34g ; proteins 13.2g; Cholesterol 106mg; Sodium :216mg

Recipe #43: Instant pot Vietnamese eggplant with spicy sauce

(Total time: 30 minutes, serving: 2)

Ingredients:

- 1 tablespoon of freshly chopped basil,
- 3 tablespoons of divided vegetable oil,
- 1 sliced white eggplant,
- 1 teaspoon of minced ginger (fresh),
- 3 tablespoons of minced lemon grass,
- 1 teaspoon of minced fresh ginger,
- 1 tablespoon of crushed garlic,
- 1 tablespoon of oyster sauce ,
- 1 tablespoon of green onion (chopped),
- 1 teaspoon of white sugar.

Directions

1. Heat 1 teaspoon of vegetable oil at medium heat inside the instant pot. Add your eggplant and then cook until it becomes golden brown and soft (cook each side for about 4 minutes but make sure it does not get mushy).
2. Get a bowl and inside mix together, the remaining 2 tablespoons of vegetable oil, with the green onion, garlic, lemon grass, Ginger, red Chile, and basil. Pour this mix over the eggplant inside the instant pot and cook until the green onion has wilted (this should take 3 minutes). Stir in your oyster sauce and sugar and then cook until the flavour have combined very well – this should take some 3 minutes.
3. Release the sealed valves slowly before opening the instant pot.

Calories: 138; Total fat: 10.4g, Carbs: 6.44g, Dietary fiber; 3.5g, Sugars 1.6g ; proteins 18.6g; Cholesterol 155mg; Sodium :323mg

Recipe #44: Crab meat with Asparagus soup

(Total time: 35 minutes, serving: 6)

Ingredients:

- 1 can (10 ounce) of drained Asparagus tips,
- 1 cup of fresh spinach (chopped),
- 2 cans of crab eat (6 ounce, drained and flaked),
- 1 cup of firm tofu (diced),
- 2 tablespoons of fish sauce,
- 2 tablespoons of dried oregano,
- 1 tablespoon of oyster sauce, and
- 1 crushed clove garlic.

Directions

1. Turn on the instant pot and inside combine the asparagus with the spinach, tofu, crab meat, oregano, fish sauce, and garlic. Make sure you fill the crockpot with water until 2 inches full.
2. Cover the mix and cook for 25 minutes on high pressure while the valves are tight sealed and the pot is covered. Make sure the spinach has cooked properly and you can smell the flavour.
3. Transfer into the serving bowl.

Calories: 140; Total fat: 13.77g, Carbs: 13.3g, Dietary fiber; 4.6g, Sugars 1.88g ; proteins 26.5g; Cholesterol 202mg; Sodium :370mg

Recipe #45: The instant pot Tomato Alfredo Sauce with artichoke

(Total time: 30 minutes, serving: 5)

Ingredients:

- 1 can (15 ounce) of artichoke hearts soaked in water,
- 2 chopped tomatoes,
- 1 chopped large onion,
- 1 cup of fresh sliced mushrooms,
- ½ a cup of chopped fresh basil,
- ½ a cup of whole milk,
- 2 tablespoon of all-purpose flour.

Directions

1. Chop the artichoke hearts and then place them in the large pan of the instant pot, then thicken them with milk and flour and mix until desired thickness and consistency are met. Press the "cook" button on the pan.
2. Add the remaining ingredients, add the lid, and then shut the valve. Cook for about 10 minutes making sure the veggies are firm and tasty. Pour the cooked recipe in a bowl.
3. Cook enough of your favourite spaghetti brand inside the hot pot, and rinse before topping up with the artichoke mix (This should take about 10 minutes).
4. Serve immediately.

Calories: 210; Total fat: 15.8g, Carbs: 14.83g, Dietary fiber; 3.1g, Sugars 1.96g ; proteins 18.4g; Cholesterol 183mg; Sodium :221mg

Recipe #46: The Instant Pot Coconut Orange Rice Pudding

(Total time: 26 minutes, serving: 4)

Ingredients:

- 2 cups of unsweetened almond milk(vanilla flavoured and divided),
- 1 cup of orange juice,
- 1 cup of Arborio rice,
- ¼ teaspoon of salt,
- 1 lightly beaten egg,
- 1 teaspoon of orange extract,
- 1/3 of a cup of coconut , and
- 1 teaspoon of grated orange zest.

Directions

1. Combine ¾ of almond milk with the rice, orange juice, and salt inside the pressure cooker of the instant pot. Seal the pressure cooker and select "manual" setting with high pressure, then set the timer at 4 minutes.
2. Let the pressure of the instant pot releases itself naturally (this should take about 10 minutes), and any remaining pressure can be released with the quick-release valve.
3. Whisk the remaining milk, with the egg, and orange extract, inside a small bowl. Add half of the cooked rice and stir the mix until they are all combined well. Pour the mix into the instant pot, and select the "sauté" option, add the coconut and orange zest and cook further for 2 minutes until the egg become set.
4. Serve immediately.

Calories: 166; Total fat: 14.5g, Carbs: 11.3g, Dietary fiber; 1.75g, Sugars 1.45g ; proteins 16.3; Cholesterol 225mg; Sodium :372mg

Recipe #47: The tasty Instant pot Aromatic Lamp chops

(Total time: 60 minutes, serving: 5)

Ingredients:

- 15 lamb loin chops (3 ounces and 1-inch thick each),
- 1 tablespoon of fresh lemon juice,
- 2 slice garlic cloves,
- 1 tablespoon of soy sauce,
- 1 teaspoon of garlic powder (for added taste),
- 2 tablespoons of olive oil,
- 1 pinch of chili powder,
- ¼ of chopped fresh cilantro,
- 2 tablespoons of brown sugar,
- 2 lime wedges, and
- 1 teaspoon of freshly ground pepper (for added taste).

Directions

1. Place the lambs inside a roasting pan, before seasoning with garlic powder, garlic, sugar, chili powder, salt, sugar, and pepper. Simply drizzle the mix with the lime juice alongside the soy sauce, and olive oil before covering and refrigerating overnight.

2. Thaw for 5 minutes, then add olive oil inside the instant pot. Add the ingredients (except the lemon squeeze and lime juice). Choose "sauté" and then close with the lid before setting the time at 30 minutes). Once it is done, simply garnish by sprinkling cilantro and squeeze the lemon and lime juices over the top before serving.

Calories: 124; Total fat: 12.1g, Carbs: 8.4g, Dietary fiber; 1.85g, Sugars 1.11g ; proteins 18.97g; Cholesterol 132mg; Sodium :242mg.

Instant pot Whole 30 Dinner recipes

Recipe #48: Sauté navy beans artichoke

(Total time 20 minutes: serves: 4)

Ingredients:

- 1 can of marinated artichoke hearts (quartered and drained),
- 6 tablespoons of olive oil,
- 2 minced garlic cloves,
- ½ teaspoon of freshly ground black pepper,
- ½ a teaspoon of salt , for added taste,
- ½ a teaspoon of ground red pepper,
- 1 can (15 ounces) of rinsed and drained navy beans,
- ¼ of a cup of grated Romano cheese

Direction

1. Open the instant pot and add the oil, set the option at "sauté", and set timer at 5 minutes at high pressure. Close the lid heat olive oil inside the instant pot and stir in the red pepper and garlic.
2. Mix in the beans and continue cooking until it becomes crispy. Mix in your artichoke hearts and then cook further for about 2 minutes before seasoning with the black pepper. Top up with Romano cheese before serving

Calories: 126; Total fat: 11.9g, Carbs: 7.6g, Dietary fiber; 3.65g, Sugars 1.8g ; proteins 10.06g; Cholesterol 104mg; Sodium :217mg.

Recipe #49: The Greek Orzo stuffed pepper

(Total time: 40 minutes, Servings 4-5)

Ingredients

- 4 yellow medium bell peppers,
- ½ cup whole wheat orzo,
- 15 ounce of rinsed chickpeas,
- A tablespoon of extra virgin olive oil,
- Chopped medium onion,
- 6 ounces of chopped baby spinach,
- A tablespoon of fresh oregano,
- ¾ cup of crumbled feta cheese,
- ¼ cup of sun-dried tomatoes,
- A tablespoon of cherry vinegar,
- ¼ teaspoon of salt.

Direction

1. Cut the pepper into halves, lengthwise, and remove the seeds. Place the cut pepper in a microwave dish, then add water and cover and microwave for about 8 minutes.

2. Pour a cup of water into the instant pot, set option at "Boil", then set timer at 20 minutes, at high pressure, then boil with the orzo inside, and then drain. Marsh the chickpeas until they turn to a paste.

3. Heat oil inside the instant pot for 5 minutes, add onion and cook for about 3 minutes, add the spinach and then stir the orzo inside, along with the chickpea and other ingredients, cook for about a minute before sharing on the pepper halves, and serve with the remaining feta.

Calories: 105; Total fat: 14.3g, Carbs: 9.6g, Dietary fiber; 1.88g, Sugars 2.07g ; proteins 11.2g; Cholesterol 103; Sodium :287mg.

Recipe #50: The Instant pot salsa chicken

(Total time: 40 minutes, serving)

Ingredients:

- 1 lb. of frozen , skinless and boneless chicken breasts (halved),
- ½ a cup of salsa,
- 1 (an ounce) pack of taco seasoning mix, and
- ½ a cup of low sodium chicken broth.

Directions

1. Place the chicken breasts inside the instant pot, then spray the taco seasoning to the sides of the chicken. Pour the salsa and chicken broth on the top.
2. Cover the pot with the lid, and choose the poultry setting before setting the timer at 15 minutes. Once the cooking has ended, simply allow the pressure to release itself naturally (this make take up to 20 minutes). Shred the cooked chicken immediately before serving.

Calories: 222; Total fat: 15.8g, Carbs: 9.7g, Dietary fiber; 2.6g, Sugars 4.1g ; proteins 23.1g; Cholesterol 281mg; Sodium :420mg.

Recipe #51: Delicious Egg scrambles with spinach

(Total time: 25 minutes, serving: 3)

Ingredients:

- 1 chopped onion,
- 3 tbsp. of peanut oil,
- A pound of lean ground beef,
- A pound of drained, chopped spinach,
- 1 tsp. of Tabasco sauce,
- 4 lightly beaten eggs, and
- 4 tablespoons of grated parmesan cheese.

Direction:

1. Heat the peanut oil inside the Instant pot for 5 minutes; add the onion and sauté until soft. Add the beef and with a fork, break the beef in pieces.
2. Cook the meat for 10 minutes and add the spinach, then mix well and cook further for 3 minutes before adding salt. Mix the egg with the Tabasco, and pour the mix over the beef mix, before cooking and stir until the eggs are set. Remove from instant pot by pressing the pressure release.
3. Transfer the mix to a platter and sprinkle the parmesan.

Calories: 155; Total fat: 14.7g, Carbs: 6.7g, Dietary fiber; 4.3g, Sugars 2.3g ; proteins 8.1g; Cholesterol 121mg; Sodium :367mg.

Recipe #52: Instant pot Rosemary Lemon chicken

(Total time: 54 minutes, serving: 4)

Ingredients:

- 6 breast halves of chicken (with bones),
- ¾ of a whole lemon (peeled and sliced into rounds),
- ½ of a whole orange (peeled and sliced into rounds),
- 3 cloves of roasted garlic,
- ½ teaspoon each of salt and ground pepper,
- 1 ½ tablespoons of olive oil ,
- 1 ½ teaspoons of agave syrup ,
- 1 splash of red wine,
- 1 splash of white wine,
- ¼ cup of water,
- 2 sprigs of fresh rosemary (stemmed).

Directions

1. Place the chicken inside the instant pot then toss in the rounds of lemon, orange, and garlic, before seasoning with salt and pepper. Drizzle the olive oil on the top, alongside the agave. Add the red and white wines, then cover with water. Add the rosemary before you put the cover lid and lock the cooker in place.
2. Select the "meat and stew" settings at high pressure and then set the timer at 14 minutes. Cook the chicken until it is no longer pink at the bones and allow the instant pot to release its pressure naturally (this should take about 20 minutes).
3. Serve immediately.

Calories: 175; Total fat: 16.9g, Carbs: 12.56g, Dietary fiber; 2.02g, Sugars 3.99g ; proteins 22.1g; Cholesterol 265mg; Sodium :417mg

Recipe #53: The 15 minute barbecue chicken soup

(Total time: 20 minutes serves: 4)

Yield: 4

Total time: 20 minutes

Prep time: 6 minutes

Cook time: 14 minutes

Ingredients:

- 2 tablespoons of extra virgin olive oil,
- 1.5 cups of chicken broth,
- ½ cup f barbecue sauce,
- 1 tablespoon of minced garlic,
- ½ a teaspoon of Kosher salt,
- 1 can of drained Mexican corn,
- 2 large cooked and shredded chicken breasts
- ¼ teaspoon of black pepper,
- ¼ teaspoon of garlic salt, and
- ¼ cup of fresh and chopped cilantro leaves

Directions

1. Add all your ingredients into the instant pot, and cover with the lid before you close the pressure valve. Then set the time at 14 minutes at high pressure.
2. Once the cooking time has been completed, simply turn the instant pot's valve off and pour soup in a serving bowl.

Nutritional Information per serving

Calories: 108; Total fat: 7.5g, Carbs: 6.3g, Dietary fiber; 0.3g, Sugars 1.86g: proteins 12.1g; Cholesterol 57mg; Sodium: 424mg

Recipe #54: The Lentils and spinach mix

(Total time: 1 hour , Servings: 2-3)

Ingredients:

- 1 tbsp. of vegetable oil,
- 2 halved and sliced onions,
- 3 cloves of minced garlic,
- ½ cup lentils,
- 2 cups of water,
- 10 ounce , or a pack of frozen spinach
- 1 tsp. of ground cumin,
- 1 tsp. of salt,
- 1 tsp. of freshly ground pepper for some taste, and
- 2 crushed cloves garlic.

Direction:

1. Add the oil into the instant pot, and sauté the onion for 2 minutes until it turns golden, then add the garlic and sauté further for 1 minute. Add lentils and water to the sauce pan, and let the mix boil , then cover an lower the heat and let it simmer for 15 minutes further when the lentils have soften.
2. Cook the spinach in microwave, then add the cooked microwave, salt, and the cumin to the pan containing lentils, then cover and simmer for 10 minutes, then add the pepper before serving.

Calories: 125; Total fat: 8.1g, Carbs: 3.8g, Dietary fiber; 1.66g, Sugars 2.5g ; proteins 10.06g; Cholesterol 89mg; Sodium :217mg

Recipe #55: Artichoke in garlic and olive oil sauce

(Total time: 25 minutes serves: 2)

Ingredients:

- 2 cloves of garlic,
- 1 chopped sprig fresh basil,
- 1 can (18 ounce) of artichoke hearts – quartered and drained,
- 3 tablespoons of butter,
- 2 ½ tablespoons of extra virgin olive oil , and
- 4 ounces of small uncooked seashell pasta.

Direction

1. Lightly salt 2 cups of water and pour it inside the instant pot and press the "boil" option at high pressure, then close the lid and secure the valve, and bring it to boil. Add the seashell pasta, and cook for about 10 minutes until it becomes dense, then drain.
2. Remove the boiled pasta.
3. Heat the olive oil and then melt the butter inside the sauce pan at high pressure (2 minutes), then mix in the garlic basil and artichoke hearts before cooking for 5 minutes, until it becomes heated through. Toss it with the cooked pasta before serving.

Calories: 96; Total fat: 15.5g, Carbs: 17.2g, Dietary fiber; 2.38g, Sugars 4.2g ; proteins 12.4g; Cholesterol 85; Sodium :262mg.

Recipe #56: Porridge served with Cinnamon

This is a delicious fat-burning aid recipe that works best in the morning.

(Total time: 20 minutes, serves: 1)

Servings: 1

Ingredients

- 30g of whole oats,
- 1 cup of water,
- ½ cup of skimmed milk, and
- 5g of Cinnamon.

Direction

1. Measure out the porridge and place in a non-sticky pan, add the milk and water before bringing to boil, turn down the heat low and let it simmer for about 5 minutes. Stir the mix to avoid one part getting cooked and the other not cooked. Sprinkle your cinnamon on top and enjoy.

Recipe #57: Arctic char with a bed of kale

(Total time: 30 minutes, servings: 3)

Ingredients

- A teaspoon of extra virgin olive oil,
- A thinly sliced large shallot,
- A cup of chicken broth
- ¼ cup of water,
- 1 pound of chopped kale,
- A pound of skinned arctic char,
- ¼ teaspoon of salt,
- ¼ teaspoon of freshly ground pepper,
- ¼ cup of sour cream (with zero or reduced fat),
- 2 teaspoons of horseradish,
- A tablespoon of fresh dill and
- 4 lemon wedges for garnishing.

Direction

1. Set your instant pot at "sauté", at high pressure, and set timer at 10 minutes, then cook shallot until soften. Add the kale and cook for 5 minutes extra, until tender. Sprinkle the fish with salt and pepper and

2. Place on the kale, cover and cook for about 7 minutes. Meanwhile, add the sour cream, dill and horseradish inside a bowl then serve with the fish, kale and the sauce with lemon garnish.

Calories: 144; Total fat: 13.6g, Carbs: 9.5g, Dietary fiber; 10.05g, Sugars 9.5g ; proteins 18.5g; Cholesterol 2174mg; Sodium :310mg

Recipe #58: The Mediterranean Fried Cabbage served with Bacon and onion

(Total time: 35 minutes; 1-2)

Ingredients:

- 7 thin slices of bacon,
- 2 tbsp. of butter,
- A small thinly sliced onion,
- A small cabbage head (cut into half),
- 2 tbsp. of cider vinegar,
- 1 optional bay leaf, and
- A cup of water.

Direction:

1. Cut the bacon into 1-inch pieces and place them in the instant pot and cook until they are ready to be turned, then add the butter and onion, and then cook until slightly brown. Add the cabbage and bay leaf, and add sufficient water to cover. This should take 10 minutes
2. Allow the mix to steam, stir and then add some water to loosen brown bits in the pan. Cook for 20 minutes, until it has attained the right tenderness. Add the vinegar and stir for 5 minutes, then sprinkle the black pepper and serve immediately.

Calories: 128; Total fat: 10.3g, Carbs: 5.8g, Dietary fiber; 1.88g, Sugars 3.04g ; proteins 9.7g; Cholesterol 136mg; Sodium :298mg.

(Preparation time: 27 minutes, Servings: 2-4)

Ingredients:

- Large Hash brown potatoes,
- 1 tsp. of pepper,
- Half sliced onion,
- 1 teaspoon of olive oil ,
- ½ tsp. of salt,
- 1 large egg
- ¼ cup of chicken broth,
- A cup of fat-free milk, and

Direction

1. Add your potatoes into the instant pot along with some oil then press "sauté" at high pressure for 10 minutes. Sauté the new potatoes, alongside the onions, pepper, then season with pepper and stir the mix until it turns brown (total cooking time should be about minutes).

2. Add the chicken broth, and cover for 3 minutes. Whisk together a whole egg, and the non-fat yoghurt. Pour the egg mix into the chicken broth.   Cook the entire mix for 15 minutes and serve immediately.

Calories: 97; Total fat: 12.7g, Carbs: 6.8g, Dietary fiber; 2.07g, Sugars 1.55g ; proteins 12.5g; Cholesterol 106; Sodium :277mg.

Recipe #60: The Red snapper Caribbean recipe

(Total time: 25 minutes, servings: 2)

Ingredients:

- A medium chopped onion,
- 2 tablespoons of olive oil,
- ½ cup of chopped red pepper,
- ½ cup of stripped carrots,
- A minced clove garlic,
- ½ cup of dry white wine,
- ½ a pound of red snapper fish fillet,
- 1 large chopped tomato,
- 2 tablespoon of non-fat feta cheese,

Direction

1. Turn on the instant pot and set timer at 5 minutes at high pressure, then Heat olive oil. Add the onion, carrots, garlic and red pepper before you sauté for about 10 minutes. Then add the wine before boiling further and pushing the veggies to one side.

2. Arrange the fillets in a single layer at the center of the pan, then cover and cook for about 5 minutes. Add the tomato and olives before topping with cheese, then cook with the fish further for 3 minutes until they are firm. Transfer the mix to a serving platter and garnish with pan juices and veggies.

Calories: 160; Total fat: 13.8g, Carbs: 12.4g, Dietary fiber; 1.7g, Sugars 0.78g ; proteins 7.5g; Cholesterol 117; Sodium :141mg

Recipe #61: The steamed-cooked artichoke

(Preparation time: 30 minutes, serving: 2)

Ingredients:

- 2 large , and whole artichokes,
- 1 garlic clove,
- 1 tablespoon of lemon juice, and
- 1 bay leaf

Direction

1. Cut and discard the stem of artichoke, and ensure the bottom of the artichokes are flat. Likewise, cut the top 1 inch of the artichokes and discard, and the thorny end of each artichoke leaves must be snipped with a scissors, and disposed.
2. Fill up the bottom of instant pot with water, and add all the ingredients.
3. Place the artichokes inside the Instant pot and make sure the artichokes rest on their flattened bottoms.
4. Cover the pot, then set timer at 20 minutes at high pressure before closing the lid and secure the valve. Bring the water to boil. Cook the artichoke until it become easy to pull their leaves away. This should take less than 30 minutes.

Calories: 125; Total fat: 8.1g, Carbs: 3.8g, Dietary fiber; 1.66g, Sugars 2.5g ; proteins 10.06g; Cholesterol 89mg; Sodium :217mg.

(Total time: 20 minutes, serving: 2-3)

Ingredients;

- 15g of Flora pro-active margarine,
- 1 medium peeled garlic clove,
- 100g of wiped and peeled mushroom,
- Philadelphia soft cream cheese ,
- 1 medium sliced Warburton bread (sliced), fresh parsley for garnish, and
- 1 pinch of salt and pepper for taste.

Direction:

1. Place half of the margarine into the instant pot, and then set instant pot at high pressure and 1 minute. Choose "sauté" option and close the lid. Add your garlic, and then cook the mixture for about 1 minute before adding the sliced mushroom.

2. Cook the mix over a low heat for about 7 minutes. Add your cream cheese and cook further for 3 minutes, and let the cream cheese melt completely into the mushrooms before you season with salt and pepper.

3. Toast your bread and spread the margarine over it, and then cut them into triangles (4), before using the spoon to spread the garlic mushroom over them. Garnish the delicious meal with the fresh parsley and serve immediately.

Calories: 140; Total fat: 8.9g, Carbs: 2.4g, Dietary fiber; 2.04g, Sugars 1.89g ; proteins 9.77g; Cholesterol 137mg; Sodium :314mg

Recipe #63: Artichoke Tetrazzini

(Total time: 25 minutes, Servings: 4)

Ingredients:

- 1 pack of linguini pasta (8 ounce),
- 1 cup of fresh sliced mushroom,
- ¼ of a cup of chopped onion,
- 2 tablespoon of butter,
- 1/8 teaspoon of dried thyme,
- 2 tablespoons of all-purpose flour,
- 1 can (10.5 ounce), of condensed chicken broth,
- 1 cup of half – and –half cream,
- 1 can (6 ounce) of marinated artichoke hearts,
- ¼ of a cup of grated parmesan cheese.

Direction

1. Open the instant pot, and opt for "boil" option and set timer at 5 minutes and cook the linguini in hot and salted water, over medium heat.
2. Once the cooking of the linguini is completed transfer it to another plate or bowl, then change the instant pot to "sauté" option and sauté the onion with the mushroom, butter, and thyme, for 5 minutes before stirring in the flour. Stir in the chicken broth plus the half and half cream, and take it back to instant pot and choose "boil" option with 10 minutes, and boil until the sauce boils and becomes thicken. Strain the artichokes and stir in the liquid into the sauce before adding the parmesan cheese.
3. Drain the linguini and toss with the sauce. Fold in the artichokes before serving.

Calories: 219; Total fat: 14.2g, Carbs: 6.4g, Dietary fiber; 3.4g, Sugars 3.8g ; proteins 22.6 g; Cholesterol 228mg; Sodium :342mg.

Recipe #64: The fresh tomato Salsa

(Total time: 10 minutes, Serving: 2)

Ingredients

- A cup of diced tomatoes,
- 1/3 cup of diced onions,
- ½ clove minced garlic,
- 2 tablespoons of Cilantro,
- 1/3 teaspoon of chopped Jalapeno peppers,
- ½ teaspoon of lime juice, and
- A pinch of cumin.
- Avocado

Direction

1. Mix all the salsa ingredients and refrigerate in advance, then coat the instant pot with oil spray, then set it at "sauté", at high pressure. Then sauté the onion and peppers lightly (6 minutes).
2. Add the peppers to your tortillas, then fill them with the pepper, onion, avocado, and salsa, then, fold the tortillas and top up with the Cilantro before serving.

Calories: 74; Total fat: 9.5g, Carbs: 8.4g, Dietary fiber; 2.1g, Sugars 0.6g ; proteins 7.9g; Cholesterol 121mg; Sodium :152mg

Recipe #65: Chicken with Artichoke and tomatoes

(Total time: 35 minutes, servings: 6)
Ingredients:

- 2 tablespoon of olive oil,
- 1 can (4 ounce) drained and sliced ,
- 1 teaspoon of salt,
- ½ sliced onion,
- 2 cloves of minced garlic,
- 1 lb. of skinless , boneless, chicken breast (cut into halves and 1-inch piece each),
- ½ teaspoon of freshly ground pepper,
- ½ teaspoon of dried basil,
- ½ a teaspoon of dried oregano,
- 1 pack (12 ounce), of Angel hair pasta,
- 1 pack (8 ounce) crumbled feta cheese,
- 1 jar (6 ounce) of sun-dried tomatoes drained and cut into quarters,
- 1 can (15 ounce) of quartered artichoke hearts(not drained),
- ½ a cup of chicken broth.

Direction

1. Inside the instant pot simply heat olive oil by choosing "sauté" option at high pressure and set the timer at 10 minutes. Add onion and garlic, and stir while cooking for about a minute extra. Add the chicken, then cook and stir for about 5 minutes until the chicken is no longer pink. Stir in the artichoke heart, chicken broth and all other ingredients then cover the skillet and simmer until the chicken is cooked thoroughly (5 minutes). Once the cooking is done simple release the valve before transferring the recipe into a bowl.

2. Get a lightly salted water inside the instant pot and boil for 5 minutes at high pressure, then cook the angel hair pasta in the boiling water while stirring occasionally until it has cooked through . Drain and transfer the pasta unto a platter and then spoon the chicken mix on top of the pasta. Sprinkle the feta cheese on top before serving.

Calories: 204; Total fat: 16.3g, Carbs: 4.2g, Dietary fiber; 1.85g, Sugars 1.6g ; proteins 17.5 g; Cholesterol 175mg; Sodium :217mg.

Recipe #66: Garlic sautéed artichoke

(Total time: 30 minutes, Servings: 4)

Ingredients:

- 2 large artichokes (about 1 lb. each),
- 3 cloves of chopped garlic,
- 2 tablespoons of butter.

Direction

1. Rinse the artichoke under cold water, then make use of a sharp knife to cut the top 1/3 part while trimming the stem to about an inch. Remove the smaller leaves located around the base, and then make use of a scissors to remove the remaining leaf tips. Cut each of the artichokes into halves from bottom to top, and make use of a spoon to scrape the hairy choke. Rinse once again to remove any leftover hairs.

2. Open the instant pot, set the timer at 5 minutes and choose "sauté" option, at high pressure. Pour the butter inside, melt the butter, before adding the garlic and then sauté for about a minute further in order to flavour the butter. Arrange the artichokes with the cut side facing down in the instant pot. Sautee the mix for about 10 minutes until they turn lightly brown, and pour ¼ of a cup of water, before covering.

3. Let the mix steam for about 10 minutes until artichoke becomes tender.

4. Once the final cooking time has been completed, simply release the valve and pour the meal in a serving bowl.

Calories: 114; Total fat: 9.8g, Carbs: 7.9g, Dietary fiber; 2.77g, Sugars 1.95g ; proteins 11.36g; Cholesterol 116mg; Sodium :301mg.

Recipe #67: The Vegetarian Cassoulet

(Total time 40 minutes, serving: 1-2)

Ingredients:

- 2 tbsp. of olive oil,
- 1 large onion,
- 2 peeled and sliced carrots,
- 1 pound of dry navy beans (soaked overnight),
- 4 cups of mushroom broth,
- 1 cube of vegetable bouillon,
- 1 small or medium bay leaf,
- 4 sprigs of parsley,
- 1 sprig of fresh rosemary,
- 1 sprig of chopped fresh lemon thyme,
- 1 sprig of fresh savoury, and
- 1 large peeled and cubed potato.

Direction:

1. Simply heat some oil in the instant pot, then add the onion and carrot inside the oil and stir until they become tender.

2. Combine the ingredients inside a pan and add water, then add to the instant pot cooker. Make sure you tie the rosemary, parsley, thyme, and savory to the pot, Stir in your potato and cook further for 30 minutes at high pressure, but remove the herbs before serving.

Calories: 88; Total fat: 12.9g, Carbs: 6.7g, Dietary fiber; 1.19g, Sugars 5.8g ; proteins 12.6g; Cholesterol 112; Sodium :219mg.

Instant pot Whole 30 Snacks and appetizer recipes

Recipe #68: The Instant pot Chinese Braised Beef Shank

(Total time: 1 hour Servings: 4)

Ingredients

- 1 lb. (454g) of beef shank,
- 1 ½ (375ml) of Chinese master stock.

Direction:

1. Clean the beef by bringing about 1.5 liters of water to boil and then boil the beef shank for 3 minutes inside the instant pot. This will help clean and remove excess fat faster.
2. Pressure-cook the beef by placing the ingredients inside the instant pot and then close the lid and set timer at 35 minutes press natural release after cooking.
3. Let the beef chill then submerge it in the master stock before chilling for 4 hours (or chill overnight).
4. Lice the beef thinly and garnish it with green onion before serving.

Calories: 118; Total fat: 18.4g, Carbs: 2.6g, Dietary fiber; 3.1g, Sugars 2.6g ; proteins 22.6g; Cholesterol 215mg; Sodium : 178mg.

Recipe #69: The Lifesaver BBQ Pressure Chicken Wings

(Total time: 10 minutes, servings: 8-10 wings)

Ingredients:

- 8-10 chicken wings,
- 2 teaspoons of olive oil,
- 4 drops of your favourite chicken wings.

Direction

1. Add your sauce to the chicken wings and make sure you marinate all over them, then pour olive oil inside the sauce pan.
2. Pressure-cook the chicken for 10 minutes inside the olive oil, while the sauce pan is covered.
3. Pat the chicken wings dry, and serve.

Calories: 94; Total fat: 9.07g, Carbs: 2.44, Dietary fiber; 1.72g, Sugars 1.08g ; proteins 11.6 g; Cholesterol 108mg; Sodium :333mg.

Recipe #70: Instant pot Avocado and Tunas Tapas

(Total time: 20 minutes, serving: 4)

Ingredients:

- 1 can (12 ounces) of packed white tuna – drained,
- 1 dash of balsamic vinegar,
- 1 tablespoon of mayonnaise,
- ½ teaspoon of black pepper (for added taste),
- 3 thinly sliced green onions, for garnishing,
- 1 pinch of salt,
- ½ chopped red bell pepper, and
- 2 ripe halved and pitted avocados.

Direction

1. Get a small to medium size bowl and inside mix the mayonnaise with the tuna, green onions, red pepper and balsamic vinegar.
2. Season the mix with garlic and salt before packing the avocado halves with the Tuna mix.
3. Garnish with the green onions, with a dash of black pepper before you pour them inside the instant pot and sauté at 15 minutes at high pressure. Then press the release manually.
4. Serve immediately.

Calories: 113; Total fat: 18.5g, Carbs: 3.8g, Dietary fiber; 1.2g, Sugars 2.3g ; proteins 14.2g; Cholesterol 220mg; Sodium :324mg.

Recipe #71: The Buffalo Chicken Scalloped Potatoes

(Total Time: 20 minutes, Servings: 4)

Ingredients

- ½ a cup of ranch dressing,
- ¼ of a cup of red hot sauce ,
- 8 red potatoes ,
- 2 cups of cooked shredded chicken,
- 2 cup of shredded sharp cheddar cheese.

Direction

1. Mix the ranch dressing with the hot sauce inside a bowl and then slice the red potatoes into ¼" thickness.
2. Pour ½ cup of water into the bottom of the instant pot, then layer the ingredients with the half of the potatoes at the bottom, followed with 2 tablespoons of the ranch sauce, half of the chicken , ½ of a cup of shredded cheese, an then repeat the layers once again. Cover the instant pot and set at high pressure for 5 minutes. Press the quick release once the cooking is done.
3. Transfer the potato mix into a shallow baking dish. Top up with the remaining ranch dressing and the remaining shredded cheese. Broil inside the oven for 5 minutes until the cheese becomes bubbly and browned.
4. Serve immediately with the hot sauce.

Calories: 123; Total fat: 14.8g, Carbs: 3.8g, Dietary fiber; 1.7g, Sugars 2.3g ; proteins 15.6g; Cholesterol 107mg; Sodium :314mg.

(Total time: 45 minutes, servings: 4)

Ingredients:

- 1 rack (2 lb.) of back black ribs (kalbi marinade),
- 1 peeled and grated Asian pear,
- 1 whole minced garlic (37g),
- 1 minced small or medium onion ,
- ½ a teaspoon of minced ginger,
- 1 teaspoon of freshly ground pepper,
- ½ a cup of light soy sauce,
- 2 tablespoons of honey,
- 2 tablespoons of brown sugar,
- 2 tablespoons of unseasoned rice vinegar,
- 2 tablespoons of sesame oil
- 2 stalks of finely sliced green onions (for garnish),
- 1 tablespoon of toasted sesame seed

Direction

1. Make your Kalbi marinade by cutting the onion and Asian pear into bits, then process the garlic and onion, alongside the Asian pear and ginger inside a food processor. Get a small bowl and inside, mix the soy sauce, with honey, ground black pepper, brown sugar, rice vinegar and sesame oil, then add the mix into the food process to create a paste.
2. Marinate your baby back ribs by removing the outer membrane from the ribs, then place the ribs inside the Kalbi marinade inside a large Ziploc bag. Close the bag partially, then marinate the ribs inside the refrigerator for about 30 minutes.
3. Cook the marinated baby ribs inside the instant pot by pouring everything from the Ziploc bag into the pressure cooker, then close the lid and set cooking time at 20 minutes (you may reduce the cooking time to 16 minutes if you want it to be more tender and chewy).
4. Turn on the heat and press the release once cooking is done. Brush the sides of the ribs and garnish with green onions and sesame seed before serving.

Calories: 151; Total fat: 16.8g, Carbs: 10.3g, Dietary fiber; 2.4g, Sugars 2.7g ; proteins 14.7g; Cholesterol 122mg; Sodium :382mg.

Recipe #73: The Instant pot cheese cake

Yield: 8

Total time: 3 hours 48 minutes

Prep time: 30 minutes

Cook time: 40 minutes

Ingredients:

- ¾ of a cup of crushed graham crackers,
- 2 2/3 of a cup of white sugar,
- 1 teaspoon of ground cinnamon,
- 3 tablespoons of melted butter,
- 2/3 of a cup of sour cream,
- 2 large eggs (stored at room temperature),
- 1 zested lemon,
- 1 teaspoon of vanilla extract,
- ¼ of a teaspoon of kosher salt,

For the batter, you need 2 packs (8 ounce) of cream cheese stored at room temperature.

Directions

4. Pulse the Graham crackers, alongside 2 teaspoons of white sugar, and cinnamon, inside the food processor, then pour in the butter, and pulse again until fine crumbs are formed. Pat the crust unto the bottom of 1 inch x 6 inch springform pan and set the pan in the freezer for about 20 minutes.
5. Get a medium stand mixer bowl and mix the cream cheese at low speed until it turns creamy and aerated. Add the remaining 2/3 cup of sugar, plus the salt, and mix further for about 4 minutes. Add the vanilla extra alongside lemon zest before mixing the batter for an extra 1 minute.
6. Crack 1 of the eggs into the batter, then add the remaining eggs. Mix for 60 seconds before stirring in the sour cream. Mix again until the sour cream has disappeared into the batter, then pour the mix into the crust-lined pan, and add cover with aluminum foil.

7. Pour the water unto the bottom of the instant pot, then add the trivet before lowering the filled springform pan slowly into the instant pot. Lock the lid of the instant pot into place.

8. Choose the manual setting and select "high pressure". Set the cooking time at 40 minutes, and allow the pressure to ease itself naturally after the cooking time. Remove the lid and check the edge and center of the cake for doneness (they should jiggle gently when shaken).

9. Transfer your cheese cake into the refrigerator and let it chill for about 2 hours or overnight.

Nutritional Information per serving

Calories: 240; Total fat: 25.8g, Carbs: 16.3g, Dietary fiber; 3.7g, Sugars 11.2g ; proteins 17.1g; Cholesterol 386mg; Sodium :450mg

Recipe #74: The Steel Cut Oats

(Total time: 30 minutes, Servings: 2-4)

Ingredients:

- 1 cup of steel cut oats,
- 3 cups of water,
- 2 slices of apples or Cinnamon(toppings)

Direction

1. Combine the steel cut oats with water inside the instant pot, then seal the valves and set the timer at 3 minutes at high pressure.
2. Once cooking is completed, let it release its pressure naturally (this will take about 20 minutes). serve the recipe with your preferred toppings

Calories: 108; Total fat: 14.6g, Carbs: 6.1g, Dietary fiber; 2.3g, Sugars 3.5g ; proteins 7.9g; Cholesterol 94; Sodium :110mg.

(Total time: 20 minutes; Servings: 4-8)

Ingredients:

- 1 ½ cup of Chinese master stock (or Chinese marinade),
- 4-8 hard or soft boiled large eggs.

Direction

1. Boil your mater stock by placing the master stock inside the instant pot, and close the lid before setting cooking time at 10 minutes. Perform a quick release once the cooking time is completed, and then open the lid gently. Pour the master stock inside a bowl and let it cool.
2. Pressure-cook the eggs by placing a steam basket inside the instant pot, add a cup of running water into the pot before placing the eggs inside the steamer basket. Close the lid and set time at 5 minutes. Open the lid after cooking and place the eggs in an ice bath for about 5 minutes and carefully remove the shells.
3. Infuse the flavour by placing the eggs into a warm bowl of the Chinese master stock, then cover the eggs before placing them in the refrigerator for 2 hours (at least), to allow the eggs soak into the flavour.
4. Serve the eggs either cold or warm inside a sauce pan, after heating for a minute.

Calories: 61; Total fat: 11.2g, Carbs: 1.7g, Dietary fiber; 0.5g, Sugars 1.2g ; proteins 12.8g; Cholesterol 75mg; Sodium :302mg.

Recipe #76: Instant pot Lentil Sloppy Joes

(Total time: 40 minutes, Servings: 2-3)

Ingredients:

- 2 peeled and diced carrots,
- 1 minced small onion,
- 2 cup of rinsed green lentils,
- 1 cup of water,
- 4 cups of pureed tomatoes (2 x 14.5 oz.),
- ½ a cup of maple syrup,
- ¼ of a cup of apple cider vinegar,
- 2 teaspoons of salt,
- 2 teaspoons of cumin,
- 2 teaspoons of dry mustard,
- 2 teaspoons of garlic powder, and
- 1 teaspoon each of chili powder and paprika.

Direction

1. Mix all the ingredients inside the instant pot, then stir very well to blend and incorporate the flavour. Cover and set time at 20 minutes before cooking at high pressure. Let the pressure releases naturally after cooking (this should take roughly 10 minutes).
2. Serve the lentil recipe with your homemade rolls, rice or potatoes.

Calories: 88; Total fat: 12.9g, Carbs: 6.7g, Dietary fiber; 1.19g, Sugars 5.8g ; proteins 12.6g; Cholesterol 112; Sodium :219mg.

Recipe #77: The Huevos Endiablados

(Total time: 25 minutes, Servings: 6)

Ingredients:

- 6 large eggs,
- 1 tablespoon of Dion mustard,
- 1 can of tuna (4 ounce, drained and packed in oil),
- 1 teaspoon of garlic (minced),
- 2 tablespoons of diced red onion,
- ½ a teaspoon of soaked paprika (you can have more for garnishing),
- 1 teaspoon of mayonnaise, and
- ¼ of a teaspoon of salt.

Direction

1. Place the eggs inside the instant pot and cover with sufficient water, bring the egg to boil over at high heat, and press quick release before removing the boiled eggs. Let the eggs remains standing in hot water for about 15 minutes before you cool them under running water, and peel.
2. Slice each of the egg into half (lengthwise), and remove the yolks before placing them inside a bowl. Get the egg white on a platter, then mash the yolk alongside the tuna, mayonnaise, red onion, paprika, Dijon mustard, and salt, until the mix become smooth and   well combined. Fill each of the egg white half with a tablespoon of the filling, and garnish with remaining smoked paprika.
3. Serve immediately.

Calories: 120; Total fat: 13.1g, Carbs: 3.6g, Dietary fiber; 4.1g, Sugars 2.8g ; proteins 12.7g; Cholesterol 228mg; Sodium :291mg.

Recipe #78: The Duck Bite

(Total time: 30 minutes, servings: 8)

Ingredients:

- ½ of a cup of dry sherry,
- 2 duck breast halves (skinned and boned),
- 1 tablespoon of soy sauce
- 16 drained whole water chestnuts,
- 1 tablespoon oil of peanut,
- 8 slices of halved bacon,
- 1 teaspoon of fresh ginger root (minced),

Direction

1. Whisk the sherry along with the ginger, and peanut oil, inside a mixing bowl, then cut the duck breast into 16 pieces and place them into the marinade alongside the water chestnut, they toss for coating. Set this aside for about 5 minutes.
2. Set the instant pot at "sauté" option at high pressure, for 10 minutes.
3. Drain and discard the marinade of the duck breast, then place each piece on a water chestnut before wrapping it with a slice of bacon. Secure each wrap with a tooth pick before placing them into the instant pot. Repeat this step for the remaining ingredient.
4. sauté until the bacon has become crispy and turn once (10 minutes)

Calories: 127; Total fat: 16.8g, Carbs: 3.3g, Dietary fiber; 2.26g, Sugars 1.2g ; proteins 17.3g; Cholesterol 140mg; Sodium :227mg.

Recipe #79: Instant pot Gambas Pil-Pil (The Chilean Prawns)

(Total time: 20 minutes; Servings: 6)

Ingredients:

- 10 cloves of garlic (slightly crushed and peeled),
- 3 tablespoons of brandy or pisco,
- ½ a teaspoon of salt,
- ½ a cup of grapeseed oil or olive oil,
- 1 ½ lbs. of large shrimp (de-veined and peeled),
- ½ teaspoon of cayenne pepper
- 1 Cacho de Cabra pepper (or Anaheim pepper), it must be seeded and cut into ½ inch pieces, and
- 1 lime (cut into wedges)

Direction

1. Turn on the instant pot, and place the garlic cloves and the grapeseed oil, and set timer at 10 minutes at high pressure. Cook until the garlic cloves turn golden brown, and the oil has become hot.

2. Add the shrimp and stir until they are coated in oil. Make sure you cook for about 15 seconds before stirring in your Chile pepper. Cook further until the shrimp has become firm and pink. Pour in your Pisco, and cook for about 30 seconds until the alcohol has evaporated. Season with salt to taste, before pouring the mix into a serving plate. Serve the meal with sprinkled cayenne pepper and garnish with lime wedges.

Calories: 136; Total fat: 12.6g, Carbs: 4.2g, Dietary fiber; 2.5g, Sugars 2.1g ; proteins 10.07g; Cholesterol 96mg; Sodium :303mg.

Recipe #80: Instant pot Pipirrana (The Spanish Potato Salad)

(Total time: 35 minutes, servings: 6)

Ingredients:

- 6 large eggs,
- 1 can of drained Tuna (5 ounce),
- ½ a cup of green olives with some anchovy or pimento (halved),
- 6 peeled and cubed potatoes,
- 1 green bell pepper (halved , diced and seeded),
- ¼ of a cup of extra virgin olive oil,
- 2 tablespoons of white vinegar (distilled),
- 1 red bell pepper (diced and seeded),
- ½ chopped large onion,
- 1 teaspoon of salt,
- 1 large chopped fresh tomato.

Direction:

1. Open the instant pot and place an egg inside, cover it with cold water before you bring the water to boil, once boiled, remove from heat and let the egg stand inside for about 12 minutes. Remove the egg and cool before peeling. Cut the eggs into quarters and set on one side.

2. Get a cup of salted water and bring it to boil in the instant pot then add the potatoes before cooking them until they become tender- this should take some 15 minutes. Drain the potatoes and transfer them unto a large bowl.

3. Toss the potatoes with the egg, and other ingredients, then refrigerate before serving cold.

Calories: 148; Total fat: 16.5g, Carbs: 4.1g, Dietary fiber; 3.22g, Sugars 5.2g ; proteins 14.6g; Cholesterol 131mg; Sodium :231mg.

Recipe #81: Instant pot Espicanas con Garbanzos (Spinach with Garbanzos beans)

(Total time: 25 minutes, Servings: 4)

Ingredients:

- 1 tablespoon of extra virgin olive oil,
- 1 can of drained garbanzo beans,
- 4 cloves of minced garlic,
- ½ a teaspoon of cumin,
- ½ of diced onion,
- ½ teaspoon of salt, and
- 1 box of frozen and chopped spinach (10 ounce of thawed and drained spinach).

Direction

1. Open the Instant pot , and heat the olive oil at high pressure , then cook the garlic and onion inside until they turn translucent(this should take about 5 minutes), with the sauté option.
2. Stir in your spinach, garbanzo beans, salt, and cumin, then use the stirring spoon to mash the beans as the mix start cooking (this should take about 15 minutes)
3. Press the pressure release and transfer into the serving bowl).

Calories: 128; Total fat: 14.6g, Carbs: 6.1g, Dietary fiber; 4.03g, Sugars 3.1g ; proteins 17.22g; Cholesterol 182mg; Sodium :267mg.

Recipe #82: The Instant pot sautéed marinated shrimp

(Total time: 30 minutes, Servings: 6)

Ingredients:

- 1 cup of olive oil,
- 2 teaspoons of dried oregano,
- ¼ of a cup of fresh parsley (chopped),
- 1 teaspoon of salt,
- 1 juiced lemon,
- 1 teaspoon of ground black pepper,
- 2 tablespoons of hot pepper sauce,
- 2 pounds of large shrimps (peeled and de-veined with the tails still attached),
- 3 cloves of minced garlic,
- Skewers, and
- 1 tablespoon of tomato paste.

Direction

1. Get a mixing bowl, and inside, mix the olive oil with the parsley, hot sauce, lemon juice, tomato paste, salt, black pepper, and oregano. Make sure you reserve a small amount for the basting that will be done later. Pour the remainder of the marinade into a big re-sealable plastic bag, alongside the shrimp, then seal and marinate the mix inside the refrigerator for about 2 hours.
2. Turn on the instant pot and set the timer at 20 minutes and choose "sauté". Thread the shrimps onto the pot and piece each near the tail and once close to the head. Dispose the marinade.
3. Cook the shrimps for 10 minutes on each side until they turn opaque. Make sure you are basting frequently with the reserved marinade.
4. Once the cooking is completed, simply press the pressure release manually.

Calories: 110; Total fat: 11.9g, Carbs: 2.3g, Dietary fiber; 1.7g, Sugars 0.8g ; proteins 14.5g; Cholesterol 87mg; Sodium :310mg.

Recipe #83: Instant pot Potato and Prosciutto Fritters
(Polpette di Patate Fritte)

(Total time: 20 minutes, Servings: 4)

Ingredients:

- 2 large potatoes (peeled and coarsely shredded),
- 2 slices of chopped Prosciutto,
- ¼ of a cup of al purpose flour,
- ½ teaspoons each of ground black pepper and salt,
- 1 large egg, and
- 1 1/4 of a cup of extra virgin olive oil

Direction:

1. Get a medium bowl and inside, place the shredded potatoes alongside the flour, egg and the ham, then mix very well. Season the mix with the salt and pepper, before forming the mix into fritters.
2. Heat oil inside the sauce pan, then fry the fritters until they turn golden in colour (this should take about 5 minutes on both sides).
3. Press the quick release once frying is completed, then serve.

Calories: 141; Total fat: 12.7g, Carbs: 2.7g, Dietary fiber; 1.8g, Sugars 3.6g ; proteins 11.6g; Cholesterol 107mg; Sodium :301mg.

Recipe #84: The Patatas Bravas

(Total time: 40 minutes , Servings: 2)

Ingredients:

- 2 russet potatoes (peeled, and sliced into 1-inch cubes),
- 1 clove of finely chopped garlic,
- 2 cups of olive oil,
- 1 minced red chile,
- 1 tablespoon of salt,
- ½ teaspoon   of smoked paprika,
- 3 tablespoons of olive oil,
- 1 can of drained whole peeled tomatoes,
- 1 diced large onion,
- ¼ of a cup of mayonnaise, and
- 1 teaspoon of salt

Direction

1. Get a large cold skillet, and inside , combine the potatoes with the 2 cups of olive oil, and 3 teaspoons of salt before heating the mix on high pressure for 25 minutes inside the instant pot and then cook until the potatoes has become softened. Dry the potatoes until they become golden in colour (this should take about 6 minutes), then drain them on paper towels after frying.
2. Pour 3 teaspoons of olive oil in the sauce pan , then set timer at 5 minutes at high pressure. Cook and stir your onions inside and add 1 teaspoon of salt inside the hot oil until the onion has been softened add the garlic, and the chile before adding the smoked paprika – simmer the mix for about 2 minutes stir in your tomatoes ad return it to simmer ,
3. Transfer the tomato mix into a blender , then cover before you pureeuntil the tomato sauce has become smooth.
4. Serve the Patatas Bravas with the tomato puree aongside the mayonnaise for dipping.

Calories: 96; Total fat: 14.6g, Carbs: 5.2g, Dietary fiber; 2.9g, Sugars 2.0g ; proteins 11.7g; Cholesterol 183mg; Sodium :208mg.

Recipe #85: The Instant pot Deviled eggs

(Total time: 30 minutes, servings: 12-16)

Ingredients:

- 6-8 eggs,
- 1 cup (250 mls) of cold water,
- 1 tablespoon of extra virgin olive oil,
- 1 teaspoon of Dijon Mustard,
- 1 teaspoon of white vinegar,
- ½ a teaspoon of Sriracha,
- 2 tablespoons of mayonnaise (full fat),
- ½ teaspoon each of ground black pepper and salt

Direction

1. Boil the eggs in the instant pot by placing the water and a steamer basket into the pressure cooker. Then place the eggs into the steamer basket before placing the basket before closing the lid. Set timer at 12 minutes and then press the quick release before opening the lid. Peel the eggs after boiling.
2. Remove the yolk from the white egg by slicing the cooled boiled eggs in halves, and remove the yolks carefully into a mixing bowl. Gently smash the egg yolks with a fork and set the egg whites aside.
3. Make the dressing by adding the mayonnaise to the olive oil, Dijon mustard, white vinegar and Sriracha, and the mix into the smashed egg yolk.
4. Pipe your dressing by placing the dressing inside a Ziploc bag and then cut a small corner with the aid of a scissors, before piping the dressing unto the egg whites.
5. Garnish your eggs by sprinkling the paprika unto the deviled eggs, and then season with the ground pepper and salt

Calories: 59; Total fat: 6.89g, Carbs: 0.85, Dietary fiber; 0.85g, Sugars 1.1g ; proteins 12.6g; Cholesterol 115mg; Sodium :285mg.

Recipe #86: Instant pot Fig and Olive Tapenade

(Total time: 30 minutes, servings: 6)

Ingredients:

- 1 cup of chopped dried figs,
- ¼ of a teaspoon of Cayenne pepper,
- 2/3 of a cup of chopped olives,
- ½ a cup of water,
- 1 tablespoon of olive oil,
- 2 cloves of minced garlic,
- 2 tablespoons of Balsamic vinegar,
- ½ a teaspoon of salt,
- ½ a teaspoon of pepper,
- 1 tablespoon of dried rosemary,
- 1/3 of chopped toasted walnuts,
- 1 teaspoon of dried thyme, and
- 1 package of cream cheese (8 ounce).

Direction:

1. Get pan and inside, mix the figs with water and place over medium heat inside the instant pot. Set the option at "boil" at high pressure and set the timer at 20 minutes. Boil and make sure the fig become tender before reducing the liquid.
2. Press quick release and stir in your olive oil, rosemary, Balsamic vinegar, cayenne pepper, and thyme. Add your garlic and olive oil and mix properly before seasoning with salt and pepper for added taste. Cover the mix and refrigerate it for about 4 hours to ensure the flavour blends very well.
3. Unwrap the cheese and place it on serving platter. Spoon the Tapenade prepared over the cheese, before sprinkling walnuts. Serve immediately with crackers or some slices of French bread.

Calories: 121; Total fat: 18.4g, Carbs: 6.22g, Dietary fiber; 3.1g, Sugars 1.9g ; proteins 19.6g; Cholesterol 118mg; Sodium :275mg.

Recipe #87: The Cheese Beer-Burger Dip

(Total time: 30 minutes, Servings: 4)

Ingredients:

- 1 cup of chopped mushroom,
- 1 finely diced large onion,
- 1 lb. of ground lean beef,
- 1/3 of a cup of beer (preferably, the Sierra Nevada Torpedo IPA),
- 1 teaspoon of salt,
- 1 teaspoon of garlic powder,
- 4 oz. of cream cheese(sliced into 8 pieces),
- 1 tablespoon of flour, and
- 1 cup of shredded sharp cheddar cheese.

Direction

1. Heat 2 teaspoons of olive oil inside the Instant pot and select "sauté". Add the beef, onion and mushrooms. Sauté the beef mix for about 4 minutes until the onion become soften, and beef starts turning dark brown. Drain the excess grease from the beef mix, and stir in the salt, and garlic powder before you pour the beer into the mix. Cover and cook for 10 minutes at high pressure inside the instant pot.
2. Press the Quick release once the cooking time is completed, then add the cream cheese, plus flour across the top of the dip and then stir to combine. Return your instant pot and sauté for about 5 minutes until the dip becomes thickened and cheese is melted.
3. Top up the dip with the shredded cheese and then cover for 5 minutes until the cheese has melted. Serve immediately with corn dips.

Calories: 113; Total fat: 17.2g, Carbs: 4.2g, Dietary fiber; 3.3g, Sugars 1.07g ; proteins 16.6g; Cholesterol 132mg; Sodium :284mg.

Instant pot Whole 30 Dessert recipes

Recipe #88: The Chocolate covered Strawberry Oats

(Total time: 14 minutes, Servings: 1)

Ingredients:

- ½ cup of strawberries,
- 1 tablespoon of mini chocolate chips,
- ¼ of a cup of boiling water,
- 1 cup of oats

Direction

1. Mix the strawberries with mini chocolate chips and mix thoroughly, then pour the water inside the instant pot. Set the timer at 10 minutes, at high pressure, then secure the valves tightly. Select "cook", and once the cooking time is completed, simply press pressure release.
2. Pour the thick and bubbly strawberry mix on your oats to coat it and cool for 2 minutes to solidify.

Calories: 132; Total fat: 11.8g, Carbs: 11.4g, Dietary fiber; 7.1g, Sugars 4.1g ; proteins 6.88g; Cholesterol 7.3mg; Sodium : 208mg.

Recipe #89: Instant pot Homemade Pumpkin puree

(Total time: 30 minutes, serving: 2-3)

Ingredient:

- 4 lbs. of pie pumpkin,
- 1 cup of water.

Direction

1. Remove stem from pumpkin. Place the rack of steamer basket at the bottom of the instant pot and add the water. Place your pumpkin on the rack or basket, and make sure the lid of the instant pot can be closed without it touching the top of the pumpkin.
2. Seal your instant pot and cook the pumpkin for 13 minutes, then let the pressure releases itself naturally. Gently lift the pumpkin out of the pressure cooker before placing it on a cutting board or plate and let it cool for about 2 minutes.
3. Slice the pumpkin in halves and then remove the seeds before you goop and peel the skin.
4. Blend the pumpkin inside a blender or food processor, and add a tablespoon of water. Make sure it is smooth after blending.
5. Store it in the refrigerator until needed.

Calories: 107; Total fat: 12.4g, Carbs: 9.85g, Dietary fiber; 8.77g, Sugars 4.7g ; proteins 11.1g; Cholesterol 54mg; Sodium : 106.4mg.

Recipe #90: Coconut little kiss (Beijinho de coco)

(Total time: 40 minutes; Servings: 10)

Ingredients:

- 1 can of sweet, condensed milk (14 ounces),
- 1 tablespoon of butter ,
- Some sweetened coconut for decoration,
- Whole cloves for decoration, and
- ¼ cup of sweetened flaked coconut.

Direction

1. Turn on the instant pot, and inside, simply bring the milk and butter to simmer over medium heat. Cook and stir continuously, until the milk volume has been reduced to half and thickened (about 20 minutes). Remove the mix from heat, and stir in the coconut and allow to cool for 3 minutes before you butter the bowl. Chill the mix in refrigerator for about 2 hours.

2. With your oiled or buttered hand, form the milk mix into tablespoon-sized balls before rolling in the coconut flakes. Decorate each beijinho with a stick of clove.

Calories: 127; Total fat: 16.8g, Carbs: 5.6g, Dietary fiber; 1.56g, Sugars 1.77g ; proteins 3.6g; Cholesterol 116; Sodium :314mg.

Recipe #91: The Toffee Almond Popcorn Balls

(Total time: 40 minutes, Servings: 16)

Ingredients:

- 2 tablespoons of unsalted butter (you may need more for shaping),
- 1 bag of miniature marshmallows (10 ounces),
- 16 cups of popped corns,
- ½ a cup of toffee pieces,
- ½ a cup of toasted almonds(chopped),
- ½ a cup of miniature chocolate chips, and
- ½ a teaspoon of coarse salt.

Direction

1. Turn on the instant pot, and inside, melt the butter over medium heat. Add the marshmallows and cook further for about 6 minutes until it melts, remove it from heat add the remaining ingredients. Once the cooking is done, simply press the pressure release manually.
2. Quickly, coat your hands with butter before shaping the popcorn mixture into balls. Place them on parchment lined baking sheet and let it cool for about 10 minutes before serving.

Calories: 148; Total fat: 12.66g, Carbs: 8.9g, Dietary fiber; 4.8g, Sugars 6.2g ; proteins 7.9g; Cholesterol 12.3mg; Sodium : 211mg.

Recipe #92: The four-ingredient toffee

(Total time: 30 minutes, Servings: 36)

Ingredients:

- 1 cup of sugar,
- 1 cup of butter or margarine,
- ½ a cup of semi-sweet chocolate chips,
- ½ a cup of finely chopped pecans, and
- ¼ of a cup of water.

Direction

1. Press the power on the Instant pot and inside, heat the butter, water and sugar inside, to boiling, while stirring continuously. Reduce heat to medium and cook further for about 10 minutes (make sure the mix does not burn).
2. Pour the toffee immediately into an ungreased cooking sheet, and spread it into ¼ inch thickness. Sprinkle the chocolate chips and let the mix stand for about 1 minute or until the chips become softened. Spread the softened chocolate evenly on the toffee before you sprinkle the pecans.
3. Let the toffee stand under room temperature for about 20 minutes and becomes firm. Break them into bite sizes an serve or store in refrigerator.

Calories: 126; Total fat: 14.1g, Carbs: 10.22g, Dietary fiber; 1.8g, Sugars 9.4g ; proteins 8.2g; Cholesterol 110mg; Sodium : 137mg.

Recipe #93: The white chocolate coffee toffee

(Total time 40 minutes, Servings: 15)

Ingredients:

- 8 ounces of white chopped chocolate,
- ½ a cup of toffee baking bits,
- 1/3 of a cup of chocolate –covered toffee bits and
- 2 teaspoons of coffee beans (finely grounded).

Direction

1. Butter a single baking sheet and line it with waxed paper.
2. Melt the chocolate inside the instant pot for 10 minutes and high temperature, then stir the mix frequently while scrapping down the sides with a spatula to prevent scorching. Stir in other ingredients and cook further for 10 minutes before removing from heat. Spread the mix unto a prepared baking dish, then refrigerate until it becomes hardened. Break them into pieces and serve.

Calories: 116; Total fat: 10.64g, Carbs: 8.33g, Dietary fiber; 5.2g, Sugars 7.9g ; proteins 9.6g; Cholesterol 82mg; Sodium : 117mg.

Recipe #94: Instant Pot Apple Crisp

(Total time: 13 minutes serving: 1-2)

Ingredients

- 5 medium to large apples (peeled and chopped into chunks),
- 2 teaspoons of cinnamon,
- ½ a teaspoon of nutmeg,
- ½ a cup of water,
- 1 tablespoon of maple syrup,
- 4 tablespoons of butter,
- ¾ of a cup of rolled oats (old fashion),
- ¼ of   cup of flour,
- ¼ of a cup of brown sugar, and
- ½ a teaspoon of salt.

Direction

1. Place the apples at the bottom of the instant pot then sprinkle the cinnamon and nutmeg. Top up with the water and syrup.
2. Get a bowl and inside, melt the butter then mix the butter with flour, oats, flour, salt, and brown sugar, then drop this mix in spoonful, on the apples.
3. Secure the instant pot lid, then make use of the manual setting and set at high pressure with 8 minutes cooking time.
4. Make use of natural release and let crisp sit for about 3 minutes.
5. Serve while it is warm, and you can top up with vanilla ice cream.

Calories: 112; Total fat: 8.2g, Carbs: 5.1g, Dietary fiber; 6g, Sugars 3.2g ; proteins 4.9g; Cholesterol 2.4mg; Sodium : 145mg.

Recipe #95: The Hard toffee

(Total time: 30 minutes, Servings: 14)

Ingredients:

- 1 cup of caster sugar (220g),
- 10g of butter,
- 2 tablespoons of boiling water ,
- 2 tablespoon of vinegar,
- 2 cups of crushed nuts

Direction

1. Turn on the Instant pot, mix all the ingredients (except the nuts), and heat on low heat until sugar dissolves, then bring to boil further for 15 minutes without stirring.
2. Pour the mix inside the paper baking cases in patty pan hole before sprinkling the crushed nuts on top. Let it set for about 10 minutes before you break into pieces and serve.

Calories: 107; Total fat: 17.6g, Carbs: 7.2g, Dietary fiber; 3.7g, Sugars 7.5g ; proteins 10.6g; Cholesterol 9.5mg; Sodium : 255mg.

Recipe #96: The Instant pot Apple sauce

(Total time: 20 minutes, servings: 10)

Ingredients

- 6-8 large or medium size apples,
- 1 cup of clean water,
- 1-2 drops of essential oil (cinnamon), and
- 1 teaspoon of cinnamon (organic)

Direction

1. Cut the apples into chunks, and throw away the stems and seeds. Place them in instant pot along with water, and close the lead before setting the instant pot at manual high pressure, at 8 minutes. Make sure you seal the steam vent.
2. The instant pot should take 8 minutes to reach high pressure, and once the timer has gone off, let the cooked apple sit for about 3 minutes , then turn the steam vent in order to release the pressure then open the lid.
3. Remove any excess water, and with the aid of electric mixer, smoothen the apple sauce to the desired consistency.

Calories: 86; Total fat: 7.4g, Carbs: 3.8g, Dietary fiber; 5.7g, Sugars 1.4g ; proteins 5.1g; Cholesterol 1.2mg; Sodium : 165mg.

Recipe #97: Carrot cake Oats

(Total time: 20 minutes, Servings: 1-2)

Ingredients

- ½ a cup of shredded carrots,
- 2 tablespoons of raisins,
- ¾ teaspoon of cinnamon ,
- ½ a cup of oatmeal, and
- ¼ of a teaspoon of pumpkin pie spice.

Direction

1. Put the oatmeal inside the instant pot and add ½ a cup of water and set at pressure cooking. Set timer at 10 minutes and secure the valves.
2. Add the cinnamon, shredded carrots and pumpkin pie spice after cooking and cook further for 5 minutes. Add the raisins to thicken the solution and let it cool until it becomes a cake.

Calories: 108; Total fat: 10.05g, Carbs: 9.4g, Dietary fiber; 4.5g, Sugars 4.7g ; proteins 12.8g; Cholesterol 86mg; Sodium : 133.7mg.

(Total time: 1 hour 10 minutes, servings: 2)

Ingredients:

- 3 cups of apple (peeled, cored and cubed),
- 1 cup of white sugar,
- 2 large eggs,
- 1 tablespoon of vanilla,
- 1 tablespoon of apple pie spice,
- 2 cups of flour,
- 1 stick of butter,
- 1 tablespoon of baking powder,

For topping, you need the following ingredients;

- 1 stick of butter,
- 2 cups of brown sugar,
- 1 cup of heavy cream, and
- 2 cups of powdered sugar.

Direction

1. Inside the mixer, simply mix the cream with the eggs, apple pie spice, butter and sugar until the mi become smooth and creamy. Stir in the apples, and then find another bowl where you will mix the flour and baking powder. Add the flour mix unto your wet mix (add half of the flour mix at a time), as the batter thickens, simply pour it into a 7" springform pan. Place the trivet inside the bottom of the instant pot plus a cup of water, then place the pan on the trivet. Set the instant pot manually at high pressure and set timer at 70 minutes. Once the timer is reached, simply perform a quick release and then remove the top with the icing.

2. For the icing, simply melt the butter inside a small saucepan, then add the brown sugar and boil for about 3 minutes and until the sugar has melted. Stir

in your heavy cream and continue cooking for about 3 minutes, until it becomes slightly thicken. Remove the saucepan from heat and let it cool before mixing in the powdered sugar and whisk until the creamy mix has no lump.

Calories: 126; Total fat: 11.6g, Carbs: 10.8g, Dietary fiber; 5.4g, Sugars 11.2g ; proteins 5.8g; Cholesterol 4.9mg; Sodium : 165mg.

Recipe #99: The Knack toffee

(Total time: 45 minutes, Servings: 48)

Ingredients:

- ¾ of a cup of light molasses,
- ¾ of a cup of heavy whipping cream,
- 2 teaspoons of cocoa powder (unsweetened),
- ¼ of a cup of chopped almonds,
- 1 teaspoon of vanilla extract, and
- ¾ of a cup of white sugar.

Direction

1. Mix all the ingredients (except vanilla extract and almond), inside the instant pot and bring the mix to a boil (20 minutes). Stir in the vanilla and almond.
2. Spoon the candy into some small paper candy cups, then cool it to room temperature before you store in air-tight container at room temperature.

Calories: 150; Total fat: 8.9g, Carbs: 7.6g, Dietary fiber; 4.8g, Sugars 10.11g ; proteins 8.5g; Cholesterol 92mg; Sodium : 218mg

Recipe #100: Instant Pot Mini-Lemon Cheesecakes

(Total time: 18 minutes Servings: 6)

Ingredients:

- 6 half-pint mason jars,
- 16 oz. of cream cheese(at room temperature),
- ½ a cup of sugar,
- 1 teaspoon of flour,
- ½ a teaspoon of vanilla,
- ¼ of a cup of sour cream (at room temperature),
- 1 tablespoon of lemon juice,
- 1 lemon zest,
- 3 medium to large eggs,
- 1 jar of lemon curd,
- ½ a cup of raspberries (optional), and
- 1 ½ cups of water.

Direction

1. Get a large mixing bowl, and inside beat the cream cheese with the sugar, and flour, until mix has become creamy and has no lumps. Beat in the vanilla, lemon juice, sour cream, and lemon zest and mix them very well. Beat in an egg at a time, and until well-mixed (do not over-beat the eggs).
2. Fill each of the jar with ¼ of a cup of the batter of cheesecake, and then drop 1 tablespoon of lemon curd on top of the batter. Add an additional ¼ of a cup of cheesecake batter to each jar and on top of the lemon curd before you cover each jar loosely with foil.
3. Add the water to the bottom of the instant pot, and ten place the trivet at the bottom. Arrange 3 of the jars at the bottom of the instant pot, and then stark the remaining 3 jars on top of the bottom three. Secure the instant pot lid and ensure that the vent remains in the pressure cooking point.
4. Set timer at 8 minutes and manually cook. Once the cooking is completed, simply perform a manual pressure release and carefully remove the jars from the instant pot with the aid of a pad or towel. Cool the cheesecakes at room

temperature until they are ready to be served.

5. Garnish the cheesecakes with raspberries and additional lemon curds.

Calories: 147; Total fat: 15.3g, Carbs: 10.22g, Dietary fiber; 6.1g, Sugars 8.8g ; proteins 13.4g; Cholesterol 107mg; Sodium : 227mg.

Recipe #101: The Butter-Pecan Fudge

(Total time: 30 minutes, Servings: 64)

Ingredients:

- 1/2 a cup of butter,
- ½ a cup of brown sugar,
- ½ a cup of white sugar,
- 1/8 teaspoon of salt,
- 1/2 cup of whipping cream,
- 1 teaspoon of vanilla extract,
- 2 cup o confectioners' sugar,
- 1 cup of pelicans (chopped)

Direction

1. Combine all ingredients (except vanilla extract and confectioners' sugar), and bring the mix to boil inside the instant pot, while stirring until the butter and has melted and the sugar has dissolved. This should take some 5 minutes.
2. Remove the mix heat then add the vanilla extract and mix very well. Stir in the confectioners' sugar, until the mix become smooth. Fold the pecans into a fudge.
3. Pour the fudge into a prepared pan and cool until it become firm (1-2 hours), then cut into 1-inch squares and serve.

Calories: 126; Total fat: 10.3g, Carbs: 6.6g, Dietary fiber; 7.3g, Sugars 8.8g ; proteins 7.6g; Cholesterol 127mg; Sodium : 107mg.

Recipe #102: The Mason Jar Steel cut oats in Pressure cooke

(Total time: 25 minutes, servings: 1)

Ingredients:

- ½ a cup of steel cut oats,
- 2 tablespoons of pure maple syrup,
- 2 tablespoons of chia seeds,
- ½ a teaspoon of salt,
- ½ cup of extras (nuts, coconut, fresh or dried fruits, and spices),
- 1 cup of water (at room temperature).

Direction

1. Add the oats, chia seeds, syrup, salt, and extras into a pint-size mason jar, then add water (while leaving ½ an inch of head space). Shake the mix until everything is well distributed and the chia seeds are not clumping together.
2. Place a small rack at the bottom of the instant pot and then pour a cup of water into the pot. Choose "high pressure" and set timer at 20 minutes. Turn off the instant pot once cooking is completed, and make use of the natural release. Remove the lid once the valves have dropped.
3. Remove the jars from the pot and place them on cooling rack. Remove the lid of the jar carefully and stir the oats very well before topping it up with a dollop of frozen whipped cream as garnish.

Calories: 98; Total fat: 11.35g, Carbs: 9.6g, Dietary fiber; 5.3g, Sugars 9.2g ; proteins 11g; Cholesterol 51mg; Sodium : 184mg.

Recipe #103: Peanut Butter Banana Oats

(Total time: 20 minutes, Servings: 2)

Ingredients

- ½ of a cup of chopped bananas,
- ½ a cup of water
- 1 tablespoon of peanut butter,
- 2 tablespoons of honey or maple syrup , and
- 1 cup of oats.

Direction

1. Add all the ingredients (except the oats and honey) into the instant pot. Then press pressure cook, and set timer at 15 minutes). Once cooking is done, simply release the pressure manually and pour the paste-like solution on top of the cooked oatmeal.
2. Add the horny and stir to achieve a much better consistency.

Calories: 88; Total fat: 12.6g, Carbs: 5.7g, Dietary fiber; 4.4g, Sugars 5.1g ; proteins 10.6g; Cholesterol 21.2mg; Sodium : 179mg.

Recipe #104: Lemon Blueberry Oats

(Total time: 20 minutes serving: 2)

Ingredients

- 1 lemon (Zest and juice),
- ½ a cup of blueberries,
- ½ a cup of oats,
- ½ a teaspoon of cornstarch.

Direction

1. Add the oatmeal into the instant pot with ½ cup of water and cook at high pressure for 10 minutes. While the oatmeal is cooking, simply place the blueberries in a saucepan, add 2 tablespoons of water, and sprinkle ½ a teaspoon of cornstarch. Stir the mix and then bring it to boil.
2. Simmer the mix and let it thicken into a syrup-like substance. Once the oatmeal is done, simply stir and swirl in scoops of blueberry and serve.

Calories: 114; Total fat: 11.9g, Carbs: 6.5g, Dietary fiber; 5.7g, Sugars 7.4g ; proteins 11.2g; Cholesterol 59mg; Sodium : 182.6mg.

Recipe #105: Lia's butter toffee

(Total time: 40 minutes, Servings: 18)

Ingredients:

- 16 ounces of melted butter,
- 16 ounce of granulated sugar,
- 3 ounces of water,
- 1 teaspoon of salt,
- 1 teaspoon of vanilla extract,
- 16 ounces of a mix of toppings (toasted nuts, sea salt, and candy canes), and
- 24 ounces of tempered dark chocolate (melted) - for coating.

Direction

1. Turn on the instant pot and inside mix the butter with the sugar, and water and bring to boil while stirring constantly (5 minutes)
2. Remove the mix from heat before adding the vanilla and combine very well. Pour the mix into a silicone baking mat or a parchment paper. Make use of a spatula to spread the toffee quickly before it sets. Spread the toffee thin and allow it to cool and blot to remove excess oil at the surface. Coat the surface with half of the melted chocolate and sprinkle with the topping.
3. Once the chocolate has set, flip over and coat the other side with the remainder of the chocolate. Sprinkle the remaining toppings. Allow it to set before breaking into pieces, and serve.

Calories: 141; Total fat: 13.3g, Carbs: 11.02g, Dietary fiber; 4.1g, Sugars 8.1g ; proteins 6.6g; Cholesterol 93mg; Sodium : 118mg.

Recipe #106: The Sri Lankan style milk toffee

(Total time: 48 minutes , Servings: 25)

Ingredients:

- 2-4 teaspoons of butter,
- 1 ½ cup of white sugar,
- 3 tablespoons of water,
- 1 can of sweetened condensed milk (10 ounce),
- ½ a cup of cashew nuts (finely chopped),
- 1 teaspoon of vanilla extract ,
- 2 drops of rose extract (for added taste)

Direction

1. Put on the instant pot , and inside, combine the sugar , butter , and water and heat at medium heat (cook and stir the mix until the sugar dissolves). Pour in the condensed milk, then cook further until milk starts to generate bubbles (about 5 minutes). Reduce the heat to low and add the cashews before you cook further while stirring frequently until the mi thickens (this should take roughly 10 minutes).

2. Stir in the remaining 2 tablespoons of butter, rose extract, and vanilla extract into the mix, then cook for about 10 minutes until the mix become stiff. Pour the cooked mix into a pan, and with a spatula or back of spoon, simply spread evenly.

3. Cool the toffee trifle until it becomes firm (for about 15 minutes), cut them into 1-inch pieces before transferring into an air-tight container.

Calories: 121; Total fat: 10.3g, Carbs: 7.4g, Dietary fiber; 7.4g, Sugars 5.8g ; proteins 8.6g; Cholesterol 76mg; Sodium : 214mg.

Recipe #107: The delicious family Almond Roca

(Total time: 25 minutes, Servings: 24)

Ingredients:

- 1 large grated and divided chocolate bar,
- 2 cups of white sugar,
- 1 lb. of butter,
- 1 pack of sliced almonds (divided and chopped).

Direction

1. Line a baking sheet with aluminum foil, then sprinkle ½ of the chocolate plus ½ of the almonds on the prepared baking sheet.
2. Turn on the instant pot and inside melt the sugar along with the butter over low heat. Increase the heat to medium and stir continuously until the mix has attained boiling(20 minutes)
3. Pour the butter and sugar mix over the chocolate and almond on baking sheet. Sprinkle the remaining almond and chocolate over the butter and sugar mix. Cool the mix to room temperature, and refrigerate for about 1 hour before breaking them into pieces, and serve.

Calories: 99.2; Total fat: 9.5g, Carbs: 4.7g, Dietary fiber; 3.9g, Sugars 4.8g ; proteins 6.3g; Cholesterol 63mg; Sodium : 204mg.

Conclusion

I want to thank you again for downloading this book!

I hope this Instant pot recipe guide has helped you learn that Instant pot recipes can be super tasty, fast and nutritious. It should also guide you through the process of retain more nutrients in your food as result of high-pressure cooking.

The next step is to jump right into the cookbook by making healthy and smart Instant food choices to ensure you meet your recommended daily nutrition and save lots of cooking time.

We have seen the immense health benefits of cooking with Instant pot. It saves lots of time and ensure that you have plenty of recipe choices to prepare within the shortest possible time.

Now, get your apron ready and start cooking these yummy dishes that will bring back food to soul of your home. All the best!

CPSIA information can be obtained
at www.ICGtesting.com
Printed in the USA
LVHW101931030321
680491LV00024B/640

9 781953 732330